PRAISE FOR MARK

C000052946

"I have worked with Mark for many years, I have no hesitation in ___, his help and input have been invaluable. He is empathetic and insightful, and my success would not have been achieved without his help and guidance"

— John Morrison
Ex England A Rugby International
and Principal of John Morrison Wealth Management
www.johnmorrisonwealth.co.uk

"By using the NLP and Matrix Reimprinting techniques that Mark has taught me, I have become a stronger and more self-assured person both physically and emotionally. Under his guidance, I have broken down mental barriers and re-defined past memories that I now realise were preventing me from achieving my goals.

I am now taking my life forward in a positive and confident way and, though at first sceptical about carrying out the exercises at all, I practice them daily with astounding results.

Mark has taken me on an amazing journey of self realization and improvement which I would recommend to anyone wishing to transform their life for the better."

— Anne Mellor

"I was successful in passing my nurse, or non-medical independent prescribing and am finding it really useful at work. Thank you for your help, the NLP really helped me in managing my study load."

— Cynthia Mellish

"I was completely inspired by your presentation and am extremely grateful for the bounty of info you've shared."

— Erika Brodnock

PRAISE FOR **ALI CHRISTENSEN**

"Ali has worked as a volunteer counsellor for the family Support Team for one year. She offers support and counselling to bereaved people and people with a life limiting illness. She has shown passion, dedication and imagination and we greatly enjoy and appreciate her as part of our team. Ali has been 100% reliable even when she has been unwell herself and has demonstrated a great resilience in coping with her own challenges. Ali is a wonderful asset to our team and her work is highly valued by her clients and colleagues alike."

— Tracey Brailsford
Family Support Team Coordinator, Ashgate Hospice

"I've known Ali for several years now and have been on the counseling journey with her. Ali's journey, though, has been particularly arduous as Ali studied with such determination, integrity, honesty and conscientiousness whilst at the same time struggling with a very debilitating illness. Ali has a core of resilience and inner strength running through her and this is evidenced in her very real and readable book, written so passionately. At the heart of the book, it's clear to see Ali's belief in her own, and other people's, positive spirit which serves to help all of us to heed the warning signs of stress which can so often precipitate illness, and for us not to waste valuable energy on negative emotions, but rather to "work with illness" in accepting it in a mindful way, thus helping us to move through illness to a place of better health and inner peace."

— Suzie Hewitt

"From the moment we first met in a classroom at the local college with some 11 other counselling students, Ali has impressed me with a combination of drive, determination and a hint of devilment. If I had to choose one person to take on a deserted island with me it would be Ali, because despite adversity she would help us through whatever was thrown at us with a great big smile on her face. Ali lights up so many lives and yet she is so modest she would have absolutely no idea. You are one in a million Ali."

— Christina Kelley

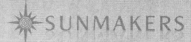

SUNMAKERS

running
away
from *ME*

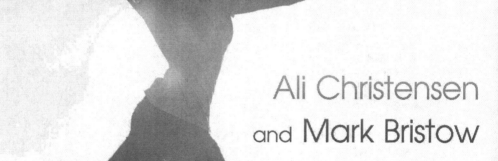

Ali Christensen
and Mark Bristow

One woman's journey
in beating chronic pain and fatigue

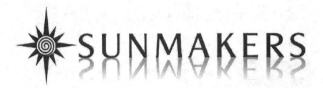

Text ©2012 Mark Bristow and Ali Christensen
Designed by Ayd Instone

Published by Sunmakers, a division of Eldamar Ltd,
157 Oxford Road, Cowley, Oxford, OX4 2ES, UK
www.sunmakers.co.uk
Tel +44(0)1865 779944

Version 1.0

ISBN: 978-1-908693-04-4

www.fusionsystemcounselling.com

To our families for all their support in this project, and
to sufferers of ME, CFS and Fibromyalgia everywhere

Acknowledgements

To Ali, for believing in me and being a willing "guinea pig"

John Seymour, all his trainers and staff and everyone on my NLP courses that helped me start on my journey to doing what I love for a living.

Karl Dawson, Sasha Allenby, Susie Shelmerdine and everyone else in "Matrix Reimprinting world" for their technical expertise, their constant support and willingness to share. You are fantastic people and it is a joy and a privilege to be a part of that world.

Peter Thomson, Steve Harrison, Jason Jackman, Sharon, Rachel, Martin, Beverly and everyone I have met on their courses. All have been totally helpful and inspiring.

And finally, my family. For their love, support and inspiration.

— Mark Bristow

Firstly I have to thank Mark. I know he hates me gushing thanks at him, but in all honesty I am not sure where I would be now if he hadn't come into my life. I will never know why he chose to help me, but he took on the challenge.

He never made me feel uncomfortable, and his patience and sense of humour made me look forward to each session, knowing I would take another small step forward. He restored my belief in myself and my recovery, and he gave me the tools I needed to get better.

We are now good friends and work colleagues, and there is no one else I would choose to work with.

I would also like to thank Savannah, and I want her to know that all the help that she gave me during my worst days did not go un-noticed. She kept my house clean, drove me everywhere, did my shopping and kept me sane. I don't know what I would have done if she had not been there for me. I love and appreciate her very much. Finally, thanks to mum for always being there

— Ali Christensen

Contents

Forewords

I met Ali in 2005 when I was working on *This Morning* as the Fitness coach and we were looking for 10 women to take part in the 'Challenge of your Life'.

All the women that applied, and there were thousands, had amazing stories, but something about Ali's story made me stop in my tracks. I can still remember her letter almost word for word.

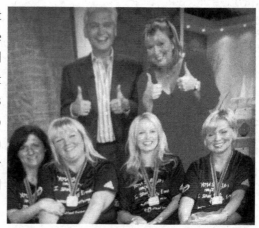

What struck me most was the lack of self pity she had. She had been at rock bottom, and I mean rock bottom, but she never once said 'Why me?' I felt that even if we didn't pick her as one of our 'challengers', she would not be knocked down, and would somehow rise like a phoenix. But there is something about Ali that shines, when she walks into a room you notice her, even though she may not be making as much noise as others. Though, don't get me wrong, I have shared many laughs with Ali! (Please don't mention my vertigo Ali!)

As I got to know Ali, I began to see many layers, and got to know her as a beautiful caring indefatigable and courageous woman. A fantastic Mum and Stepmum. She is inspirational and I am privileged to call her my friend.

— Julie Dawn Cole, Actor, TV Presenter and Fitness Coach

Forewords

I first met Ali in 2005, she had followed my story on *This Morning* and was taking part in a challenge of her own, a mutual friend introduced me to her and we got on really well. Little did I realise at the time how much Ali was going through herself.

To come through the things she has over the last couple of years is nothing short of miraculous. I regret, apart from the odd email, I have not been as good a friend to Ali as I could have been but I have been aware of some of the things she has come through I have been moved to tears by the things she has had to deal with - abuse, bankruptcy, court cases and illness - I really don't know how she is still here, a weaker person would have taken their own life by now. But she is still here and despite all this continues to help other sufferers as a counselor and believer in EFT and Matrix.

She is a true inspiration to us all - of course like us all she will have her dark days but I feel sure she, you and I will come through these days together. It is a pleasure to write a foreword to this book, it's an honour to know Ali and she confirms my belief that there is nothing that can't be overcome with a little bit of help and support. By buying this book today you have taken the first step on the road to recovery a path already started by Ali and so many of us.

— Charlie Walduck, Radio Manchester Presenter

An Introduction

This book highlights my fight to recover from Fibromyalgia (Chronic Pain) ME (CFS Chronic Fatigue Syndrome) and ultimately Depression. It explains how Matrix Reimprinting, EFT (Emotional Freedom Technique) and NLP (Neuro Linguistic Programming) helped me in that recovery.

I want this book to show people that there is hope out there for what some in the medical industry have described as incurable disease. It is so difficult for sufferers and their families to understand the origin and development of these illnesses and that in itself makes the condition worse.

There are no Fibromyalgia/ME specialists where we live in Cheshire UK, and only one nurse allocated to this illness in the Greater Manchester area. I want this book to show that there is an answer and provide the catalyst for people who are suffering from these dreadful illnesses to seek the correct help from the wonderful practitioners that are available worldwide, many of whom have suffered from the same or similar illnesses.

The book is written from a very truthful personal perspective. It starts the journey when I was extremely ill and had absolutely no idea what was wrong with me. During this time I kept a journal, partly to keep me sane and partly because I wanted to remember how bad and hopeless I actually felt.

I had been through a ten year period of immense hardship, which may seem unbelievable when reading, but is absolutely true. It included horrific abuse from my alcoholic/drug addict husband, whilst coping with my own business and financial ruin, ultimately leading to bankruptcy and losing my home. It also involved watching one of my adopted children go completely off the rails and fight a custody battle for my grandchild. Also, during this time, my oldest daughter was diagnosed with advanced cervical cancer whilst pregnant and I had to provide the support required to help save her and the baby she was carrying.

Through all of this, I managed to study and become a qualified Psychodynamic counsellor, whilst bringing up the rest of my children and putting them through university. I also held down a full time job to support everyone financially.

In the middle of 2009 after my daughter had the all clear from cancer, my body decided to pack up, and I became very ill indeed.

In spring 2010 after many tests, hospital visits and counselling, I was no nearer a diagnosis nor a cure, and I felt my life was over. It was at this stage that I saw an email from Mark Bristow advertising his technique. Having lost all hope I decided to reply and Mark brought NLP, EFT and Matrix Reimprinting into my life.

This book follows the journey from the beginning of this illness, giving in-depth descriptions of symptoms and feelings, through the first meeting with Mark and the scepticism I felt initially, to feeling at least 90% better. The book is written in the form of my diary, each one starting a new chapter. It starts in January 2010, describing the illness, treatment and personal discoveries that come from the treatment. Mark then covers each session, with his own perception on how the treatment is working and why it works. As a counselor I had worked with and experienced many types of counselling and positive thinking techniques but none that had the effect that the Matrix did. My work in this book is because I am passionate about helping others who are suffering. My experience as a counsellor, plus all the real life traumas I have endured, gives me deep empathy with fellow sufferers.

This is why I have written so much on a personal level about my pain and illness, as other books I have read on ME always seem to be written after recovery has taken place. They do not describe in detail how absolutely dreadful the patient feels. In writing this book I hope that more doctors will take notice of this condition, and more specialist centres will be set up.

– Ali

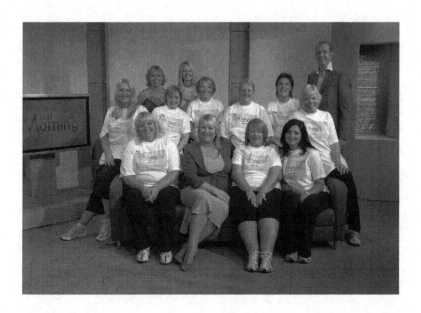

Ali on 'This Morning', front row, left.

running away from ME

1: Trying to make sense

You would think that with all my experience as a counsellor I would have the answer to all the problems in my life. However even with all that knowledge, I still couldn't fix what was happening to me, and I seemed to be on a never ending spiral down into the depths of an illness that was destroying my life.

When I got ill in the physical sense, I lost the ability to even think in a rational way and had all but given up on living all together. What I did not realise was that there were indications that I was getting ill long before I was bed bound, and if I had taken notice of the deterioration in my body, I might have been able to address it sooner and stop myself becoming so ill. They say hindsight is a wonderful thing!

The question is how much psychological stress can you put your body under before it begins to retaliate and breakdown physically? IBS, insomnia, muscle stiffness or a poor memory may just sneak up on you and unaware that they may be leading to a more sinister condition, you just carry on popping the odd pain killer to see you through.

So no matter how bad the mental pressure was, I had coped and carried on regardless.

In Buddhist medicine they believe that the body and mind are interdependent, and the health of the mind influences the health of the body and vice versa. The Buddhists seek to cure both physical and mental illness treating them as one, but emphasis is placed upon the mind. Bhuddha said all illness arose from the three poisons: Greed, Anger and Ignorance. These three negative emotions were the catalysts for many destructive emotions that eventually could manifest into physical ailments. Therefore it was not enough just to remove the physical aspect of the illness, but instead cure the mind based causes that initiated the illness to begin with.

Western medicine approaches illness through its physical symptoms. This approach tends to temporarily reduce the symptoms for a period, but the lack of symptoms does not mean that the root cause has been identified and removed. Therefore you run the risk of the disease reoccurring. And so in my case, my poor body was feeling robbed by the fact that I had not taken any time out to let my mind heal itself so it decided to rebel in such a way that I had no choice but to take notice.

One day it just decided to pack up and shouted, 'I HAVE HAD ENOUGH OF THIS, YOU (meaning my mind) ARE NOT LISTENING TO ME, SO I AM GOING TO MAKE YOU HURT, I AM GOING TO MAKE YOU SO TIRED YOU CAN HARDLY GET OUT OF BED, AND THEN I WILL NOT LET YOU SLEEP PROPERLY BECAUSE OF THE PAIN IN YOUR BACK AND LEGS. I WILL AFFECT YOUR PERSONALITY, YOUR EATING HABITS, YOUR BOWELS, YOUR MEMORY AND ANYTHING ELSE I FEEL LIKE UNTIL YOU STOP WHAT YOU ARE DOING AND LISTEN TO ME!' And so I fell victim to a disease that just made me want to curl up and die.

A depression that had manifested for many years and been left untreated was now so deep rooted now that it was accepted as a normal part of my life.

Even though on a conscious level I had accepted these negative and destructive emotions as being normal, my subconscious was not so willing to accept this and so it took action.

Fibromyalgia means widespread chronic pain, whilst ME/CFS is known as a chronic fatigue condition. Both of these conditions are very difficult to specifically diagnose, and many doctors are reluctant to make that diagnosis, mine included. I had many tests done with so many conditions thrown at me. A tumour on my pituitary gland, Cushings Disease, Polymyalgia Rheumatic, adrenal failure, thyroid dysfunction to name a few, yet none of the tests came back conclusive, and because of this I began to feel an overwhelming sense of hopelessness. The pain that enveloped my entire body was unbearable. The illness was worse, I can only describe it as being like the worse hangover you have ever had, even though you never drank a drop, and it persisted day after day after day. The exhaustion was overwhelming and this of course led to worry that in turn led to irrational thinking.

Thinking was about the only thing I could do and that manifested into a fear that there was something very sinister wrong with me, and this in turn led to panic attacks.

For those of you who have suffered from panic attacks they are extremely frightening, and death seems only round the corner. I had come across people who suffered from panic attacks during my work, but even being aware of what was happening to me did not take away the fear, nor did it enable me to get control of them. I felt defeated and totally alone.

The thought that all my symptoms were psychosomatic did not make the symptoms any less real for me. The pain and tiredness were only part of it, and those of you who are suffering now will know that everyone is individually affected in different ways. This also does not help doctors reach a clear diagnosis. Some people with ME suffer no pain yet they are chronically ill and cannot get out of bed. Their immune systems shut down and in extreme cases this can lead to life threatening illness.

It is miserable when doctors tell you they cannot find anything wrong, and you feel like no one believes you. I have broken down and sobbed in front of doctors and consultants, who seemed sympathetic but could offer me no more than repeat blood tests, pain killers and depression pills. To say I felt completely helpless is an understatement. I wanted a miracle cure, in fact I wanted more than that, I just wanted someone to tell me what was wrong with me.

It is difficult for people to understand how disabling this condition is, especially when tests results are coming back indicating there is nothing seriously wrong. Not being able to put a finger on what is wrong with you is extremely difficult to live with. To finally be given a diagnosis is like seeing your enemy for the first time. It puts things in perspective and gives you the chance to fight back. Stabbing around in the dark facing an unknown foe is a horrendous way to live. Stress is becoming a major factor in many people's lives. Everyone wants so much from us. Bills mount, kids expectations are never ending, companies we work for want every piece of you they can suck dry, whilst the banks seem to control our very existence. Maintaining standards and trying to cope with relationships in a material world can be soul destroying. Too much of everything is available to us and even relaxation time at home can be disrupted by salespeople calling you at all hours. It's exhausting and every day it starts up all over again.

Even going on holiday is no longer a 'get away from it all' experience. You still carry your mobile, visit internet cafes, and have the underlying fear that a terrorist has targeted your aircraft. The money you thought would be enough, runs out and you dare not let your children out of your sight for a minute. Sometimes walking back into your own home is a relief after it all, yet you do it all again the following year.

These are all normal everyday problems that everyone of us encounters, so god forbid that you have to endure worse and throw something else into the mix. The death of someone close, an abusive relationship, being bullied at work, bankruptcy and debt, a delinquent teenager hell bent in ruining their life and dragging you along with them, losing your job, alcoholism, watching someone go through a terminal illness or losing your home. There are more I know, but these are the ones I dealt with over the last ten years.

Add these extreme stresses to your normal amount of stress and you have a concoction that can be extremely damaging to your health.

Whilst you deal with all this on a conscious level and seemingly are coping, your sub-conscious is manically trying to handle all the stuff being thrown at it. You carry on regardless, unaware of the danger, whilst your sub-conscious is crying out to be heard.

2: The beginning of the illness

In 2006 I was picked by ITV's *This Morning* to do a Challenge of your Life. I had just left my alcoholic husband after losing our home due to his drinking. We had gone bankrupt, so I was starting out again with my kids. I felt I had something to prove and that I would not be beaten. So I threw myself body and soul into the challenge. I had to run the London Marathon and the Great Wall of China Marathon and had six months to prepare, whilst having film crews follow my every step. In doing this I completely buried the emotional pain I had felt from losing my home and the years of mental abuse I had suffered from my husband. Of course it was buried but it did not go away, so when I had finished the race and the challenge and the focus was gone, the buried emotions and feelings came back to the surface with a vengeance. I was struggling at work. I worked for Tesco as a line manager in the fresh food

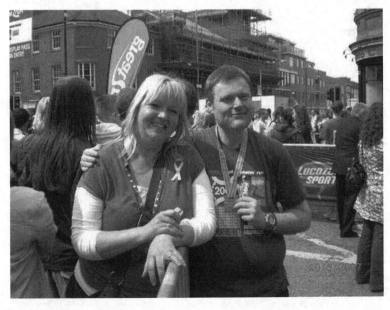

department whilst going to night school to train as a counsellor. My job was extremely active, involving lots of lifting, carrying and stretching. I enjoyed my job and got on well with all the staff there, but I would get incredibly stiff after a long shift and would hobble around. I was overweight when I ran the marathons and the trauma on my body was huge. I was virtually crippled after the London Marathon and could not move for over a week. The stiffness I was feeling after a long day's work was similar to how I had felt then.

I carried on regardless, using pain killers as a crutch. Then in 2008 my oldest daughter was diagnosed with cervical cancer and my health was put on the back burner again.

Over the following year I had a lot of time off to be with my daughter who had to have four surgeries to save her and the baby she was carrying. When she and her daughter started on the road to recovery and I could stop worrying so much, my body decided it was time to pack up.

I had gone down to stay with my daughter in Brighton when her baby came out of hospital after three months in intensive care. I was trying to help her cope with all that had happened, although I had been in a great deal of pain for months, especially in my legs and groin area, but I had ignored it. After a few days, I started to feel like I was getting flu, in fact I felt so ill I got up at 4am and drove back north earlier than planned. I did not want to risk my daughter, her partner or their baby getting ill. The drive was very difficult, I felt absolutely terrible, sweating, head thumping and when eventually I managed to get home I found I could hardly move after five hours in the car. I crawled into bed and hardly got out of it until I had to go back to work six days later.

I still felt dreadful and was in sheer agony at work, but the doctor had given me prescription painkillers. They had little effect and I still felt exhausted all the time. It became a pattern, I would go to work doped up on pain killers and diet coke hen I would drive home and go straight to bed. I worked different shifts, so I had no pattern for sleep at all and eventually I went to back to the doctor's. He thought I may have a condition known as polymyalgia rheumatica and decided to try 30 mg of steroids.

Now polymyalgia is usually a condition that affects people in their late 60's or 70's, so it is extremely rare for someone of my age to get it. However, the steroids seemed to work and it was initially like a sudden cure, the pain was gone within 24 hours and I was out of pain for the first time in years. I did not realise how much pain I was actually in until it was gone. I was so relieved, yet it didn't last long. I began to feel even worse than before. I was shaking violently all the time, my blood pressure went through the roof, and I just wanted to sleep.

I managed work as the pain was gone, but it was a struggle and on my days off I stayed in bed. I had gained a huge amount of weight in a matter of weeks and looked and felt dreadful. I went to the gym to try to get fitter. I went swimming, but I would feel worse after activity, and I was frequently calling into work sick. I began having pains in my chest and eventually extreme pains one night put me in hospital. My blood pressure was ridiculous, 210 over 170 and I was very ill. I was kept in and taken off the steroids as quickly as possible, but anyone coming off steroids will tell you it is not a quick process. This was at the end of November 2009 and I was not completely off them until January. I was written off work with Christmas coming upon us, our busiest period in the store, and I felt so guilty. By the end of December the pain had returned, but this time it was all over my body. I couldn't even bear anyone hugging me. I was put on Tremadol and co-codimol, and I went back to work just after Christmas. It was short lived, I think I managed a week, just, and then the illness just over whelmed me.

I never went back to Tesco's.

January through to March remains in a fog I was so ill, there were times during my worst days when I did not care if I lived or died. I scared myself during one of these dark spells, when I contemplated taking my own life. I knew I would never do it as I would never inflict that on my family, however I wanted to hurt myself, anything that would deflect from the illness. I even planned of getting hold of a heavy pan and smashing myself in the face with it until I had broken my nose and blackened my eyes. I could not even have gone down to the kitchen, let alone been able to lift a heavy pan, but I went through it all in my head. It was then my rational side kicked in and I knew I was really struggling mentally with this illness. The doctor started me on 20mg of cilitropan, a mild depression pill that did help a little, especially with the panic attacks.

After months of illness and seeing different consultants, with no help being offered, I explored the internet to try to find the answers. I had matched my symptoms to those of Fibromyalgia and ME, joined websites with fellow sufferers and found we had so much in common. I decided to try to find other means of a cure. I had studied Cognitive Behavioural Therapy (CBT) briefly during my course and knew that it was used as a therapy by the NHS for ME sufferers. The NHS offers six sessions of CBT which is a therapy that looks at how you are coping with life in the present. The therapist looks at different techniques that would help make your life easier and sets you homework to try these out.

In some cases CBT could be helpful, perhaps with people with obsessive disorders or a particular phobia, but I felt it would not go deep enough for me. The sessions offered would not even scrape the surface of the hidden patterns of behaviour that my subconscious had developed over years.

Also on a more realistic level, the thought of doing homework when I couldn't even hold a book was just too much. I started seeing a psychosynthesis counsellor recommended by someone on my course. Psycho synthesis was developed by Roberto Assagioli in 1911, and it looks at the different levels of consciousness and the vast human potential for healing and change. It does work on a somewhat spiritual level looking at the higher self (soul) and I hoped it would give me some insight into what I had repressed and help me to discover how deeply my feelings ran. I did discover why I had put up with Biff (my ex) for so long, and how much damage it had actually done me. However knowing the reasons still did not make me any better and after three months and a lot of money that I could not afford, as my statutory sick pay was now at an end, I decided to call it quits.

So I was back on my computer, tired and sore looking for the miracle. I was still seeing consultants, who were at that time testing me for pituitary and adrenal gland problems, but nothing was resulting in this, and they were still reluctant to tell me that I had ME.

By a fluke I was suddenly getting emails from a mind and body company. I have no idea how I got on their mailing list, but it caught my interest.

Mark Bristow is a practitioner of Neuro Linguistic Programming (NLP) and the Emotional Freedom Technique (EFT). He and his partner Ben run this company together at one of the local gyms. Their main objective is weight loss and a healthy way of living both in the mind and the body, so I emailed them to ask how I could lose weight when I could not even get out a chair and to my surprise Mark contacted me. The rest shall we say is history and what happened next is a fascinating journey that I want to share. Even if you do not pursue the same path, I know that when you are as ill as I am, it is important to know and understand your feelings and know that there are others out there that have the same feelings too.

What follows is a series of journals that I kept during my illness. Initially I wrote them to keep myself sane, but as time went on I realised that they may be a help to others who are going through similar processes. Being ill brings all sorts of other problems, such as finance, family dynamics and future planning.

This journey is about trying to find the answers and I will be totally honest about what helps and what doesn't.

My life has been extremely complicated, and I think it's fair to say that I have not discovered a quick fix to this illness. I have discovered a whole new way of living thanks to Mark, and it has improved my health greatly. As I move forward I am in no doubt that by the time this book is completed I will be mostly cured.

3: Is life worth living?

January 2010

I have never felt so ill in my entire life. My whole body hurts so much, the pain is unbelievable. I cannot even be hugged as just the touch is too much. My eyes hurt to blink, and my jaws hurt to talk and my throat is raw. I cannot lie in bed for hours as the pain in my back becomes unbearable, yet just walking to my chair is a nightmare. I sit with my neck propped up, but my body just seems to throb, even flu wasn't this bad.

My daughter comes over and helps out, bringing me shopping, and cleaning the house for me. I still manage to eat even though my jaws ache, I have a craving for sweet things all the time.

I have never felt so tired, I alternate from chair to bed, dozing in both but never getting a good nights sleep as the pain wakes me within a couple of hours. I am dosed up on co-codamol and tremadol, yet they only take the edge off. People come to visit, but I don't want to see them. I just hate the way I am and I wish people would just leave me alone. I have started having a problem trying to swallow when I lie down. I feel like I have a lump in my throat that will not go away. Then I start to panic that I will not be able to breathe and will suffocate. That's when I think I am going to die. The panic goes all round my chest and up into my head. I am gasping for air and trying to tell myself its all in my head, but I don't seem to be listening. I get up and hobble back to my chair to see if I can switch on the TV

I have told my son to leave the remote on the arm of the chair, but he forget sometimes and it's on the floor. I cannot bend down to reach it, so I just sit. I can't read as I cannot hold a book for long, my wrists are too weak. I feel so pathetic and helpless.

The doctors don't know what is wrong with me, and the tests come back showing that I should be ok. But I am not ok, I just feel defeated by life. If I have to go on living like this, then I do not want to go on living. There is no point, what use am I to anyone? Everything is so hopeless here, the kids are worried but don't know what to do. Nobody understands, because I don't understand. I have been through enough, and I feel like I am being punished again. What is happening to me?

4: Body packed up

3rd February 2010

My body has packed up! It has just stopped working and everything hurts so much. I was always so strong, there was nothing I couldn't do or achieve. I weighed around 16 stone, so I was heavy but I was so fit. I worked ten hours a day on my feet, lifting and carrying. I would spend a couple of hours in the gym then go for a long swim on my day off. I brought up five children and managed all the chores that that entailed without a thought. Three years ago I ran the London Marathon and the Great Wall of China half marathon, and now I couldn't even crawl for a bus. I found an old journal I had kept dated the beginning of 2008, just before Suzanne, my daughter got ill. The funny thing is that I was clearly suffering body pain even back then. I had stopped going to the gym because I was so exhausted on my days off. I just put it down to my job being so physical, yet I did actually have time off for a week with total exhaustion and body pain. It was totally unlike me to take time off, so I must have been bad. I had forgotten about that, and perhaps should have recognised that something was going wrong then, but I didn't. I just went back to work and carried on, always tired. I had too many other things going on in my life to notice, not least of all when Suzanne got cancer.

At 28 I never expected to become a full time mother, of four children, Suzanne (9), Katie (7), Maxine (4) and my own baby girl, Robyn. I had backpacked around the world, had many adventures and a family was the last thing on my mind. However I had met and fallen in love with a bit of a renegade American (Biff), and moved to Orange County, where I discovered he had three children living in a hell hole with their drug addict mother. After a vicious custody battle I became full time mum with sole custody.

It was easy to love Suzanne and Katie, they were so sweet. They flourished under my care and did really well at school considering they had missed so much. They suddenly had a home they could be proud of and could bring friends back to. We moved to the UK and I had another baby (Craig), and started my own catering business. My husband then discovered his love of pubs! I guess I was too busy to notice, with five kids and a full time career.

Maxine was a different matter. Nothing I could do for her ever helped. She had terrible behavioural problems from the start, to the extent I sought professional help when she was only seven. Nothing helped and she got worse as she got older. She had violent rages, told outrageous lies that caused a lot of trouble, and eventually became addicted to drugs and alcohol. I spent years blaming myself for not loving her enough, but she was so difficult. She had more than the other kids, yet it still was not enough. She became so manipulative I questioned myself at every turn. I look back now and wonder if I would have done things differently if I had known or understood these behaviours better. In a professional term now she would probably be diagnosed as having a 'borderline personality', but back then noone knew or understood what was wrong with her.

Suzanne and Katie went on to get law degrees and become successful young women, while Maxine just managed to keep herself out of prison.

Biff's alcoholism was horrendous and I could no longer hide it from my friends and family. He spent all our money on drink or expensive sporting events, boxing in Las Vegas, or Formula One races. He did not care and was extremely abusive to me all the time. I was broken by 2005, and discovered that the only way out to get away from him and everything else was to declare ourselves bankrupt.

It was probably the most humiliating and difficult time of my life, but I got through it and started to put my life back on track. I started work for Tesco and began a counselling diploma at university. It had been so hard over the years and I felt like things were changing for me, so when Suzanne phoned to tell me she had cancer in 2008 at the ripe old age of 27, I felt like the very last drop of belief I had in a better life had been sucked out of me, someone up there hated me. I was shocked beyond belief and drove straight down to Brighton where she and her partner, Luke, lived.

Everything for myself went on the back burner. For the next 14 months I lived and breathed hospitals, operations and in the end a miracle. Suzanne and Luke had been trying for children, but discovered Suzanne had a particularly nasty strain of cervical cancer. It was devastating for them and she was very low. She told me that if she couldn't have children then she did not see the point of going on. She had always dreamt of having a large family. She had her lymph nodes removed almost immediately after diagnosis, and was referred to the Royal Marsden hospital in London. They decided to try an operation called a tracholechtomy, where they would take the cervix away and attach the womb to the vagina, giving her the chance to have children. It was risky, as her type of cancer was particularly aggressive and they did not know how far it had spread. Then came another bombshell; just before they were about to go into theatre, a test revealed that she was already pregnant, against all the odds.

I have always been intuitive and as soon as they told me, I knew this baby would survive. The baby should not have been able to be conceived due to the cancer, let alone survive two previous operations. Suzanne and Luke decided to go ahead with the pregnancy although it was risky as the cancer was an aggressive strain and if she went to term it would definitely kill her. So they rearranged the tracholechtomy for when she was over three months pregnant. The operation took about six hours, but miracles do happen and the baby survived the op. She hung on in there for another couple of months but was born at 25 weeks. Little Skye was 1lb 10 oz when she was born and spent three months in hospital. It was extremely hard on everyone as there were many worrying moments, and it was difficult for Suzanne being in that baby unit every day watching other tiny babies lose their fight for life. I never had a moment's doubt that Skye would survive, but it was so hard on Suzanne and Luke, especially as the cancer growth had been larger than the consultants had anticipated, and there was some concern that it may have spread into her bladder.

During this time I was struggling more and more to walk. I would stiffen up after a couple of minutes of not moving and the pain in my legs was horrendous, however I struggled on, my mind totally focused on Suzanne and Skye.

As if that wasn't enough worry, Maxine had had a baby daughter (Alicia) 18 months before. I had spent a great deal of time helping her make a home for the baby, but to no avail and the child was taken into care when she was three months old. Max managed to get off the drink and drugs for a period and Alicia was returned to her, but it wasn't for long. She soon went back to her old ways and the poor child was removed again. During all of this I had remained in contact with Alicia and loved her dearly. I was there when she was born and had taken care of her many times. The sad thing is that Maxine did not understand how to care for a baby. Even at 22 she still behaved like a small child herself putting her own needs before her child's. Alicia's eyes were always red rimmed with exhaustion, but Max would continue to have friends round and music blaring half the night. Alicia had a permanent cold and Maxine would have her out in her buggy all the time including the middle of the night. Maxine was evicted from her house again, but of course it was the neighbours fault, not hers. Nothing was ever Maxine's fault and I just did not know what to do. I was so mortified and embarrassed by her behaviour and the way she treated people. I took it very personally and felt totally helpless. Social services told me they were going to put Alicia up for adoption.

The pain I was in daily and my lack of mobility made the thought of having to look after a toddler impossible. Suzanne and Luke decided to go for custody, but Suzanne had to get the all clear from the cancer first, so at the time it was looking unlikely. Everything was in such a mess. By August 2009, I was disabled by the pain. I lived on prescription painkillers the doctor had given me, but I hobbled like an old woman. I still worked full time and was doing a diploma at night school, but was in bed whenever I was not at work. Suzanne and Skye had come to live with me in Cheshire to recover from the past year in hospital and get to know Alicia better. She and Luke had put themselves forward to be Alicia's foster parents, with the view to adopt when they could. The doctors could not find any traces of cancer left so it was looking good. I was so tired and down and very negative thinking life was so unfair. It had been so difficult these last five years. I lost my husband to alcohol, my house to debts created by alcoholism and nearly lost my daughter to cancer. Robyn had just finished school and had gone to university and Craig had just started sixth form. I am aware that all of these events have probably led me to the place I am in now, but I wish I could be strong for my younger children's sake. Sleeping is so hard because of the pain, so I just cannot snap out of this low mood.

I don't know what is going to happen to me, and it won't be long before I will be unable to pay the rent. The kids are brilliant but I know it's really worrying everyone that I am so ill. It is not something they have seen before, I was always the strong one, the one that kept everything together.

5: Losing the will

3rd March 2010

This last six weeks has been a living hell, and I feel so hopeless.

My throat feels constantly blocked and I have panic attacks at night because I think I am going to suffocate in my sleep. I start sweating for no reason, and my hands shake really badly. During all of this I am still undergoing tests. After initially ending up in hospital in November 09 with an adverse reaction to steroids, I was referred to the Diabetes and Endocrinology Department with my first appointment being 23rd December. That was awful, the consultant was not available and I saw her registrar who was only interested in my blood pressure and did not seem to take the pain I was in seriously at all. He suggested a series of tests that would investigate my cortisol levels and I was referred to see the consultant in February. So I waited for another six weeks before I saw the consultant. The tests had come back indicating a low cortisol count, but the consultant thought the test was corrupted due to the steroids I had been on. So it was arranged for the same tests to be redone and I was given another appointment to see the consultant again at the end of March, six weeks later. The test results have now just come back and they are showing the same results as before so yet again, more tests have been organised and another appointment has been made for the end of April.

We are getting no further. I am still in terrible pain and it is very difficult to get myself to the hospital, I have to rely on my daughter. I was very depressed and my GP has put me on depression pills, 20mg of citalopram. After a couple of weeks

I started to feel like I could cope better and also the panic attacks stopped.

I have begun to notice that if I get anxious about anything then my symptoms will really worsen. Depending on how anxious I get it will affect me in different ways. If it is a minor argument with my teenage son, for example, I would have to go and lie down for a couple of hours to stop my head pounding and my body shaking.

If it is a crisis situation, which unfortunately we seem to have plenty of with the Maxine/Alicia saga, sometimes I just have to write the day or even the week off. Mum came to stay in February with all good intentions of helping me. I got so worked up because I am used to having the house looking nice and looking after her, that I became so ill during her visit that I just couldn't get out my chair. Mum was so depressed when she left, she just did not know how to help me and it was awful for her seeing me so ill. I was eventually referred to a rheumatologist. She took a number of blood tests, but thought as did the other consultant that there was something wrong with my pituitary gland and that that was the reason I was in pain, but when the blood tests came back clear, she just referred me back to the original consultant. I think the steroids have messed my system up so much that no one really knows what to do. If I had been sent to the rheumatologist in the first place, before being put on steroids, I may have had more chance of a quicker diagnosis.

This whole process is unbelievable. I went to the doctors last September in agony, I have been in pain for almost two years now and yet no one has told me what is wrong or how to fix it. I am desperate. I cannot work and am having to manage on statutory sick pay now. They have given me housing benefit, but I feel such a criminal. They ask me what is wrong and I just don't know what to say. I am becoming a recluse, and am losing touch with my friends. I feel out of control and I want to be in charge of my life again.

6: A light in the darkness

1st June 2010

I don't know how I got on his mailing list, but I was sent an email by a neuro linguistic programme/EFT practitioner. It was a newsletter that he sends out to all his clients, and he was talking about the new fusion system he had been developing using EFT and NLP.

I have no idea why I got it as I had never heard of this. It was very interesting and after doing some research I emailed him about my situation.

He replied saying that he thought he could help but then I suddenly thought better of it, as this was clearly how he made a living and I had no money. However he emailed me again telling me not to worry and asked if we could meet and I agreed.

He was called Mark, we hit it off straight away and I could tell he was on the same wave length as me. He explained to me all about NLP and the Emotional Freedom Technique, as well as a new approach he was working with called matrix re-imprinting. This is about reliving distressing and bad memories, and changing them so they become more bearable. He seems genuine and wants to give me all the treatment for free and use me as a case study. He truly believes he can help cure me and get rid of all this pain.

I am sceptical, but I have no reason not to try. So I followed his lead and started tapping myself on my head.

Yes, I know what you're thinking, but as I say I am open to most things so I sat there tapping my head, telling myself that I love and accept myself.

I guess if I hadn't have gone through so much already I would have really have thought this was weird, but Mark truly believes in this and I have the feeling that his email did not just appear by accident. He showed me the points where to tap: the top of my head, just above my eyebrow, the side and below my eye, my upper lip, my chin, my collar bone and down below my armpit where my bra strap is. This was followed by tapping on each one of your fingers. During all this tapping I would concentrate on one particular area, let's say my neck and shoulders. I would imagine the pain to go away, all the time telling myself that I love and accept myself.

After the tapping he got me to roll my eyes, hum happy birthday then count to ten. Yes I felt like a complete idiot and was glad none of my kids could see me. They already think I am barking mad and this would have given them just cause to have me sectioned.

The crazy thing is that it did work. The pain was reduced quite dramatically although it started coming back when I concentrated on it. Still I could feel the benefit so he arranged to come back next week and start working on some of my memories.

I have to admit I am curious. I have an exam to sit next week for my diploma and I have found studying so hard whilst I have been ill, but it is the only thing I have been able to focus on and when I have not made it to class my tutor has been sending me the work so that on good days I have been able to catch up. This is my final year and this course has kept me sane during all of this. I am worried about sitting on a chair for two and a half hours during the exam. I have timed when to take my painkillers so any extra help I can get will be appreciated. If I pass this exam I will have qualified as a Psychodynamic Counsellor and I cannot help but think that if this works then maybe some of my clients would benefit from it. Well it is early days yet, but I have a good feeling about this and I have been blessed with a good intuition.

Mark takes up the story:

For me I had been suffering from long term frustration, rather than long term chronic pain. When I was growing up, in my teenage years, I had this dream that one day I would make a difference in the world and leave a lasting legacy. Anyway, leaving school at 18 to pursue a 'safe' career in financial services that dream seemed to fall by the wayside as 'real life' got in the way.

Don't get me wrong, I wasn't an unhappy person, just a bit unfulfilled and frustrated that I something was missing in my life and I couldn't quite put my finger on what it was.

In the conscious world, my childhood was great. My parents were always supportive and I remember mum being the only spectator at a school rugby match when dad couldn't get there, and she didn't even know the rules! We had brilliant holidays and always had fantastic birthday and Christmas presents.

My father had missed out on a family life as his own father had worked away from home before going off to war then returning home only to die at the early age of 42. Dad therefore was determined that my sister and myself were going to benefit from family life to the full.

So I tried various jobs within the financial services industry and did ok at all of them, but nothing more. It wasn't until later that I realised why. A colleague of mine had talked about NLP (Neuro Linguistic Programming) and this seemed fascinating. I dabbled with this for a while, trying to learn it from books and buying lots of CD programmes from the Tony Robbins organisation. These were fantastic but there was still something that was missing, I was to find out what this was later.

Eventually I must have been so frustrated at myself that I enrolled on an NLP course with John Seymour. This is when my life really began to change. During a ten minute exercise which involved defining my life statement, I realised that I was in totally the wrong profession. This was all somewhat ironic as consciously I had enrolled on the course to become better at my then current job.

From that point on I realized that my mission in life is to help as many people as possible and then I set about discovering the best way to achieve it. However, the story doesn't end there. Although I had these strategies in place to achieve my dream, there was still something holding me back. This is when I met Karl Dawson, EFT (Emotional Freedom Techniques) master and creator of Matrix Reimprinting on a marketing course. Karl had demonstrated his techniques one evening and everybody was raving about how he had changed someone's life within a really short time span The marketing guys were saying that he increase his course fee twenty fold. To what I think is his eternal credit, Karl kept his fees at the same level, his goal for being on that course was about far more than making money.

After talking briefly with Karl I felt that he was the person who could provide me that missing link and so it proved. Whilst learning about EFT and Matrix it suddenly all made sense. It is, I believe, pretty much all down to this!

If your subconscious is running negative programmes about yourself, then no amount of positive conscious thinking will override this. The way to move forward in your life is to get rid of those negative emotions and to reimprint new ones. It is like when your computer is running slowly and you try to load new programmes, it won't run any better. It is not until you get rid of the viruses in your neck top computer that you can install the new beliefs and habits. Now that I had this picture in my mind of how it all worked I knew that using a combination of NLP, EFT and Matrix Reimprinting I could help Ali change her past and transform her future.

The idea of this book is not to provide a detailed explanation of the workings of Matrix Reimprinting, EFT and NLP, however, along the way I hope to give an insight into what I believe are cutting edge personal development techniques.

I would thoroughly recommend the book *Matrix Reimprinting using EFT* by it's creator Karl Dawson and Sasha Allenby. For a detailed introduction to NLP, a great book is *An introduction to NLP* by John Seymour and Joseph O' Connor. For the scientific background to EFT and Matrix, I would suggest you check out the work of Bruce Lipton and Robert Scarer

NLP (Neuro Linguistic Programming)

NLP (Neuro Linguistic Programming); Neuro being the brain and our senses, Linguistic being the thoughts and words we use for ourselves and others and Programming, how this affects your behaviour. NLP can be likened to a computer – it is programmed by the words and thoughts behind them and hence then acts in a particular way; if you know the words, language and have the skills you can reprogramme the computer to work in a way that benefits you. One of the co-founders of NLP, Judith DeLozier, indicated that NLP would be instrumental in finding ways "to help people have better, fuller and richer lives". NLP is the difference that makes the difference between excellent and average, can help in leaving behind certain aspects of your life that are holding you back, and is a way of discovering and achieving your own personal genius. It is unlike other forms of coaching as it works at a deeper level to ensure beneficial and long lasting change.

EFT (Emotional Freedom Techniques)

EFT recognizes that the majority of diseases (dis-ease) have their origins in life stresses, beliefs and traumas, and that to heal any condition we have to heal the mind and body simultaneously.

The easiest way to describe the actual process of EFT is to say it is like acupuncture but without the needles. Instead the relevant points are tapped upon by our fingers. (A more detailed explanation and a guide on how to tap can be found in on page 166 of this book)

Matrix Reimprinting

This takes the workings of EFT a stage further and was developed by Karl Dawson in 2006. It finds its basis in quantum physics which states that we are all composed of energy; furthermore, we are all connected by a unified energy field, referred to, by Max Planck in 1944, as 'The Matrix'.

Karl believes that we hold all the stressful life events that have gone before in our fields. These are held not just as memories, but as specific energy bodies, which he has named ECHOs (Energy Conscious Holograms). By working with the Echos, it is possible to resolve the negative energy charge around them. This removes the negative emotions associated with the memory, therefore improving our emotional and physical health, both in the present and in the future.

Most, if not all of our negative habits and beliefs are created within the first six years of our lives and even in-utero. At that age we have no conscious mind as such and therefore what can seem to be a fairly trivial event later on in life could lead to the formation of a negative belief. Once the belief has been created, a part of your brain called the Reticular Activating System seeks evidence to support this belief. This is essentially a filter between your conscious and your unconscious mind.

Therefore, in order to help rid someone themselves of a negative belief or habit, it is really helpful to get to the initial source and deal with the memory. EFT aims to take the emotion out of the memory where Matrix takes things a stage further and 'reimprints' a new belief.

Since my "aha!" moment during my advanced EFT training, I had been looking at how I could impact what I had learned on as many people as possible. One of the attendees, Lydia had explained how she had offered free consultations in order to promote herself. With my colleague Ben, a personal trainer, we had built up a mailing list of people to whom we provided weight loss tips on a weekly basis. I decided to use this forum to offer free consultations with a view to writing the ultimate weight loss book containing advice about how to have the correct mindset, nutrition and exercise. This is the email I received from Ali in response to my offer:

Hallo,

I have a problem and I am trying everything I can to solve it. So I wonder if your experiments and know-how can help. I am 5ft 9in and currently on scales today at 20 stone 6lbs. Morbidly obese.

In 2007 I ran the London Marathon and the Great Wall of China marathon. I weighed then 14 stone, so I was not skinny, however I was very fit. Since then I developed polymyalgia rheumatica which considering my age (47) is rare, and have been in constant pain daily. Some days too painful to get out a chair, some days (yesterday) I can walk for an hour, although painful it does make me feel better but I do pay the next day with stiffness in all my muscles.

I got put on steroids, which did a wonderful job and made me pain free. However the diverse side effects made me put on a load of weight, raised my blood pressure dramatically and made me very ill. So I was weened off, however my pituitory gland is now all messed up and my natural cortisol production is very low, and I am being investigated for Cushing's disease. I try very hard to diet and lose weight, I do not eat fatty foods, though I do have a sweet tooth, but again, I do not overload on chocolate or sweets. I am totally miserable at this weight. The pain I am in makes it very difficult to take regular exercise.

Am I doomed, or is there a solution?

I await your reply with interest regards

Ali

Now having read this, a strange thing happened. Normally I would have considered this too big a task and look to pass this on to someone else as at the time, I hadn't resolved my own issues about not being good enough. If I needed help, I didn't have to look far, After all, Sasha Allenby, who co-wrote the Matrix Reimpinting book with Karl Dawson, had suffered from ME and would be ideally suited to work with Ali.

However, something, or someone (I am hoping it was dad, who by this time had passed away) told me that I was actually good enough to deal with this. What also gave me confidence was that I had that my upmost belief in NLP, EFT and Matrix which meant that I knew that I could help Ali. I knew from reading about Sasha's experiences that it wasn't going to be a quick fix but I made a commitment to Ali and myself that I was going to be in for the long run.

I spoke with Ali over the phone and we agreed to meet up and see whether we could work together to help rid her of what she was later diagnosed as fibromyalgia.

I therefore met up with Ali and went through how I felt I could help her. I taught her basic tapping and showed how I felt this could help reduce the pain she was experiencing. Often we are the last port of call in a bid to find a cure for this type of illness and so it wasn't a total surprise that Ali wanted to take things forward and to meet up again.

7: Positive interventions

8th June 2010

I have loads to tell you, I feel quite excited about things today. I don't know where to start. The exam was quite hard and I am hoping I managed to get everything down, I was so focused that I did not notice the pain, and the time went so quickly. In fact at no time did I feel uncomfortable and it was an incredibly long time to sit in one position on a chair. I would not have been able to do that at home, so I have to ask the question, is the pain all in my mind? It was funny watching everyone else and how they handled the stress. There were 21 of us, most of us were in our 40s and had not sat an exam since school. My last exam was when I was 16 and I certainly never took them seriously then. My poor parents were so disappointed at my lack of effort and absolute lack interest in the education system.

You know? I actually enjoyed it! I did not even notice the examiner having a sign language battle with the grass blower who was outside the window, which annoyed most of the class. I was so focused I amazed myself and now I just have to see whether I pass or not. The results are not out until middle of August, so fingers crossed.

Mark came round the next day and we went to work on the first negative memory I had from my childhood.

It was when I was around six years old and Mum had taken me, my brother and baby sister to the Highland show in Edinburgh. I remember walking around the highland cattle paddocks, Mum had a pram with my sister in it. I asked if I could look at the calves and Mum told me to meet her at the other side of the long tent. We somehow missed each other and I became a lost child.

I walked around looking for Mum for a while and then thought I would walk to the car. So I walked out the grounds and although it took me a while, I managed to find our car and I sat and waited. I was very pleased with myself for finding it.

Of course inside the grounds loud speakers were calling my name, Mum was frantic and sick with worry, the people at the gate told her that no child would have walked out unaccompanied, and the police were called.

Meanwhile I was lying looking at the sky sucking the juice out of the long grass.

Eventually some people saw me and realised I was the missing girl and went to tell them I had been found. I remember seeing Mum walk towards me with the pram and a policeman with her. I expected to be told I was good for finding the car, instead mum was furious. She couldn't even speak to me, she just glared at me and threw me in the car.

I was taken home and sent to my bedroom without tea. I lay there in disgrace waiting for my dad to come home. He was furious with me and I felt like a really bad person for the first time in my life. For years afterwards we were never allowed to mention the Highland show and I would cringe if I saw the signs anywhere.

So Mark decided to work on that memory. He tapped on me while I had to use my imagination and tap on myself as a child. As he tapped he asked me to describe how I was feeling as the child. He then asked me to introduce myself as an adult to my child self. I had to imagine I was there as an adult in the situation. I then had to imagine what I would say to my child self. So I saw myself hugging me and telling me that Mum had just been really scared and that was why she was mad. I could really picture it in my head and I'm sure the tapping made it easier to concentrate. Mark then asked me to introduce someone else into the memory. So I brought in my Aunt Kathryn, who is my Mum's sister, they are very close. So I imagined her there and she was hugging my child self and telling Mum to stop being silly, she said that I was safe that it had been an accident that we missed each other and that I was not being naughty, but thought I was doing the right thing.

Mark asked me to tell him what Mum was doing. I told him she was crying and it made me feel a bit better because she wasn't angry anymore.

He then stopped tapping and suddenly asked me about the books on my bookcase. I started explaining them to him and then he interrupted and told me to think back to the memory again.

It was incredible and totally amazed me. I could not think of that trip to the Highland show without Aunt Kathryn being there and my mum crying. My whole memory of it had been altered and it was no longer making me cringe when I thought about it.

As a parent I know I would have been shaken to the core if I lost my child. I cannot even begin to imagine how terrible it would have been and now I can see it all from my mum's perspective. Before this I could not get past the awful memory of being so bad. I had no understanding of my mum's reaction. Now I can see it all and empathise completely with how frightened she would have been, it must have been just the worst feeling ever. I am now fascinated by this work, and am very keen to learn more about it. I hope to have the faith that Mark has and I know that it will help cure me.

Mark's Perspective: First Session

I spoke with Ali on the phone and we agreed to meet up and see whether we could work together to help rid her of what was later diagnosed as fibromyalgia.

The first session started with me obtaining the some background information from Ali. She has covered her story in her *Alison in Wonderland* fairy tale (see page 157 of this book) and it soon became clear that there were a number of events in her life that could have helped to contribute towards her condition. However, I felt it was important to get to the source of any major negative belief that she had about herself.

It became clear that Ali had an issue with not being good enough for her parents and in particular with her mother. We therefore worked on her particular memory of getting lost at a highland show.

Whereas Ali thought she had thought she had been sensible by going back to the car, her mother was angry with her and it was at this point that the belief was created.

I asked Ali to visualise the incident and then asked her lots of questions regarding her memories in order to bring the scene to life. It is important when using Matrix for the client to picture the scene as if they were watching a film or on TV, that is to say that they disassociate themselves from the scene. The picture that Ali had visualised was at the moment that she had been found and a particular look that her mother had given the young Ali. The young Ali is what Matrix terms an Energetic Consciousness Hologram, or ECHO. I then asked Ali to step into the picture and introduce herself to her ECHO, explain who she was, give her Echo a hug and say that she was here to help. I then asked Ali what the response was from her ECHO and she said that she was pleased that there was someone there to help her. I then asked Ali to tap on her Echo as she was upset and afterwards she said that she felt better.

One of the great things about Matrix Reimprinting is that we are able to change a particular memory and create a new positive one however we want to. I then asked Ali to ask her Echo whether there was anyone that she wanted to bring into the picture. She said that she would like her Auntie to be brought in. Her Auntie was, and still is, her mother's best friend, and would tell her mother not to be so angry with young Ali, so we got her to do this. By doing this the situation seemed to change completely as Ali's mother stopped being angry and became warmer towards her.

At this point, I asked Ali if there was any particular place that she wanted to go at this point in order to give the memory a happy ending.

I was really pleased at the way the first meeting went as Ali was able to interact with her ECHO. This is a very positive start and it boded well for future sessions. Ali's demeanor was very different after the session and whilst I detected that there was some skepticism towards this work, I felt that she would be open for more sessions. However, I wouldn't really know until I saw her again the next week.

8: Living on drugs

15th June 2010

This weekend has been shit. My back became unbearable on Friday night. I couldn't sleep at all because of the pain. I can understand why people overdose on pain killers. I have both prescription strength co- codamol and 50mg tremadol tablets. I took three co-codamol and two tremadol at once and it did absolutely nothing to take away the pain.

I wish I could drink alcohol as it might have knocked me out, but I knew it would only make me feel worse. I got up at 3.30am and sat in my broken down chair. It's so comfortable, it has a nice high back that supports my neck, but it's sinking in the middle. I sat almost the whole weekend, flicking through the TV channels. I have finished all my books and have not the energy to go and buy a new one.

The kids stayed away and I tried to do some tapping to make the pain go away. The trouble was I could not lift my arms for long, it took too much energy to tap. I gave up and wallowed in self pity.

That's when the panic sets in. I start to worry about my career and if I am ever going to earn enough money to buy a house. I wonder if I am going to be able to cope with any sort of job and negative thoughts seem to swamp me. It does nothing to aid my recovery, but being in so much pain makes it hard to focus on the positives. I feel I am going to let Mark down. He seems so excited about this all and I just feel deflated. He is due soon, so I will just sign off while he is here...

Well he has just left and has given me loads to think about. He wants to carry on changing my painful memories so I can look forward and find positive steps to move forward with life. I told him the most crucial thing for me is to get rid of the constant pain and then I would be able to walk without hobbling and perhaps start to exercise and get into shape. I do miss exercising but admit I am really disabled, even swimming is so difficult. I tried but my shoulders and arms stared to shake and I didn't know how I was going to get out of the pool.

He suggests that I may be hanging onto the pain; that as life has become so difficult for me, I use it as an excuse not to carry on. It's strange thinking that all this pain is due to something in your head and I am not totally convinced about that. However I am willing to try anything.

So the next memory we confronted was my 40th birthday. It was an awful time for me. My wonderful parents had wanted to give me a birthday worth remembering and had booked a beautiful country hotel and invited all my family and some friends for a huge dinner. They also paid for my husband and I to stay the night at the hotel while they looked after the kids.

My main concern was hiding Biff's alcoholism from them, and he was at a stage then that he didn't care how he behaved. To make matters worse he was trying to get me to sell the house, move all the kids down to Exeter and put whatever money we had left into managing a pub. Of course I said no, but he was furious and hell bent on making my life hell. Everyone had made such an effort for my birthday and he had not even bought me a card, let alone bother to acknowledge it.

The first night we were there we rowed nearly all night. He was livid and wanted his own way, and I just wanted to get through the weekend without being embarrassed. I ended up sleeping on the floor of the hotel room while he was passed out on the bed. He woke in the middle of the night, sat up and hit me a couple of time with a pillow, cursing at me. The next day people were arriving and giving me presents. I was so embarrassed when they asked what Biff had got me. I said he was surprising me later. I could see in their eyes that they didn't believe me, but my family was too classy to embarrass me further.

We got through the night and Biff kept his mouth shut for the best part, though he got very drunk. He also took himself off to bed before everyone else, which was a relief, but I knew my mother was furious with him. Again nothing was said.

I went up to bed later and he was vile to me, calling me fat and ugly, telling me my parents didn't really love me, that I was an embarrassment to them. I started to cry and he sneered at me, telling me I was a lazy, underachiever and all I could do was snivel. It was an awful night, but at least he had saved this behaviour for the bedroom, and my family didn't have to see it.

The next morning we went down to breakfast. He refused to sit with my sister and her husband, so we sat across from them. He wouldn't speak to me and I was trying to pretend that everything was ok. We left and he wouldn't let me go round to Mum and Dad's to say thank you properly. I love my family and I felt so awful that I had such a horrendous time, when they had gone out of their way to make the weekend special for me. I told Mark the story which was difficult and he decided to work on the memory. We used the same technique as last time and I went into the memory while he was tapping on my head. I told my echo (which is what we called my younger self) that everything was ok, that there was no point trying to hide his behaviour because everyone knew. I said that everyone just wanted to help me and they all loved me very much. Mark then got me to introduce someone else and I chose my old best friend Dawn. She appeared, and told my ECHO that I was going to dump this loser soon and I would never have to look back, that I was not to listen to a word he said and that I would do great things with my life. She told me that I had to learn from this so I could help others in the future who were going through the same thing. She also told me that I still was very strong and that I was not to allow him to sell our house. She then made him tired and he went to bed, and I shared a room with her that night and sat with her and my sister the next morning for breakfast.

The same thing happened as before. I no longer felt embarrassed and I stopped caring about what he had done. When we revisited the memory I saw Dawn there, and it was all ok. I don't know if revisiting all these difficult moments will help in the long run, but it does make it easier when remembering them. I no longer get that sick feeling of being ashamed, so it has to be a positive.

Mark's Perspective: Ali's 40th Birthday

The law of attraction meant that having created a belief, the universe and the Reticular Activating System will look for evidence to support it. In Ali's case she got herself a husband who was only too willing to support her belief by continually putting her down. With this in mind, I asked Ali to recall a particular occasion which felt prominent in her memory where Biff had indeed put her down.

Ali's recollection of her 40th birthday party spread over the whole weekend so I asked her to run the memory as if it were a movie and to give the movie a title (This, unsurprisingly in EFT / Matrix terms, is called the Movie Technique) Ali entitled the film "The birthday from hell".

Having run the movie, it is then important to concentrate on one scene from the movie that was the most poignant for Ali. This was during the party itself and I asked Ali to step into the picture and tap on her "Echo" and to offer words of encouragement. I also asked whether she wanted to bring anyone else in at this time, whereby she suggested her friend Dawn. I then encouraged her to run the movie in the way that she wanted, together with making her own conclusion.

Once we had completed the scene I asked Ali to open her eyes and we talked for a few seconds on an unrelated subject in order to break her state. I then asked Ali to go back into the memory and test what emotions she was now feeling.

The movie technique is one that is often used during EFT and Matrix Reimprinting sessions. The important part to this is to concentrate on one scene at a time with the client making the scene choice. It is highly possible that in the future we would be revisiting that particular movie and concentrating on another scene.

The wonderful thing about directing your own movie in this way is that you can choose how the movie ends. Furthermore, in choosing your own ending to the movie, you attach a positive belief to the experience and replace

running away from ME

the negative one that previously existed. Without doubt, changing this memory alone wasn't going to rid Ali of her belief and I felt that we were going to have plenty more memories that involved Biff, however, we were one step closer towards getting Ali back to full fitness.

9: Anxiety is the trigger

29th June 2010

Sorry, it's been nearly a couple of weeks but things are moving slowly forward I think.

I got extremely stressed the day Mark came. Mum had just phoned the night before to say she and Dad were coming to stay on the 10th July. I couldn't sleep at all worrying about sorting the house out before they came. I made myself ill, and the pain got intense. It dawned on me that my illness gets worse when I get anxious. I don't lose my temper often these days, I think I had all my temper sucked out of me during my marriage. However the other morning I discovered that Craig had not applied to Manchester college yet and when I went in his room to confront him I was met with more horror than any human being should face.

His room was in a word 'DISGUSTING' and I snapped. He jumped up and cleaned his room and we sorted out the college, however just that short exertion of temper left me shaken and exhausted. I ended up in bed.

It's like my body does not recover from any increase in adrenalin, any bad news or something to worry about knocks me for six. I know I have to get on top of this now. I think recognising this is the first stage.

I have had many tests done now and all show that I should be healthy. I saw the doctor this morning and he said "Well on the plus side at least you know you have nothing seriously wrong".

Maybe I am mad but how can that be the plus side? If I am lying in bed for a week unable to walk without being in agony and yet having to tell myself there is nothing really wrong with me it makes me doubt my sanity. I pointed this out to him. It is extremely difficult when no diagnosis is given, to move on with your life. You cannot make plans, think of work or know when you are going to get better. I need to be able to see the demon so I can fight it, but when it's invisible I can't do that.

He told me I definitely had fibromyalgia and possible ME, though it was hard sometimes to distinguish between the two. He was surprised that I didn't already know that and equally surprised when I said that would make a huge difference in how I deal with this. Now I know what I am battling, my enemy has a name, I must and can defeat it. Just to add a personal note, he did apologise on behalf of all the doctors for being 'UTTERLY CRAP' during this period. OK he didn't use the word crap, or utterly come to think of it, but I'm sure he meant it.

I have to do another series of tests over these next few weeks, but I am sure it's just so the consultant can say she has tested everything and can draw a line under my case. The 24 hour urine sample was a nightmare though. My legs were swelling so I took two water tablets before I started. You have to pee into a great big brown pot with a lid. They put some sort of acid in it to preserve the urine. Trouble was I got the pot a few days before and we were having a bit of a heat wave. All the acid had vapourised into a cloud of toxic gas. So when I took the lid off it wafted out burning my throat, lungs and eyes. I tried to pee into it holding my breath, with stinging eyes, when I felt it burning my 'hoohoo' as well. What a nightmare! To make matters worse the water tablets took effect and four hours after I had started the 24 hour test, I had filled the huge pot to the rim. I could hardly lift it.

The next test they want me to do is a 24 hour blood pressure monitoring. It's where the blood pressure device is placed on your arm and is set to go off every 20 minutes. Normally these things tighten and hurt, but try to imagine doing this with fibromyalgia when just touching my arms hurts. I have had enough, it's not my blood pressure making me hurt, it's the pain that's making my blood pressure high. I am not going to put myself through agony just so another box can be ticked. Someone has to fix this pain! Mark came today and I told him about what the doctor had said. He understood how frustrated I had been, but could see I looked much more positive about the situation. I have decided that I am no longer going to wait from each six week appointment to the next, hoping for a miracle cure. Today I have decided wholeheartedly to embrace the EFT technique and get rid of the illness. We worked a lot on the pain and created a timeline where I pointed out different changes I would make to my life to eventually reach my goal.

Work phoned and said they could retire me on ill health if they could receive a letter from my consultant. The first letter was requested in February and still they have heard nothing even though they have said they will pay. They have sent reminders as have I. This has been crippling for me financially. I cannot claim disability and my statutory sick pay has run out. All savings and shares have been cashed in and I am relying on help from my family. At least if they retire me I can use up my pension, claim disability and income support. All it needs is a letter from the doctor confirming I am too ill to work. It's another nightmare with this condition that you constantly feel that you have to justify your illness. With no accurate test results the doctor's can only take you at face value. You have to explain your symptoms over and over again. I have looked at maybe doing part time office work where I don't have to move around, but some days I feel so ill, what would I do then? I want to earn money more than anything, as I have worked all my life I'm not exactly work shy. I hate claiming benefits, but I don't know what else to do.

I feel really let down by the NHS. This process has been so long and is so difficult. It does not help with your recovery with all the added stress and tension of having to prove you are ill, when all I want to do is get better.

Mark's Perspective:

Although Ali felt let down by the NHS and that she had to jump through a number of hoops just to get any sort of diagnosis, my instincts had told me that Ali wouldn't feel she was making any real progress until she knew exactly what she was up against.

I suggested that it was a breakthrough now that there had been a definitive diagnosis of fibromyalgia.

If we are to believe that a lot of illnesses are emotionally lead, these illnesses can continue to provide negative thoughts, especially when recovery seems to be happening at a very slow pace. Now that we knew that Ali had fibromyalgia, we could forsee that it would be a longer road to recovery. This removed some of the pressure to find a 'one minute wonder' that would cure her overnight.

Logic suggests that there were a large number of experiences that Ali endured in order to generate the negative emotions that eventually resulted in her body closing down.

The problem with negative thoughts and emotions are that the more we think of them, the more new negative thoughts and emotions are generated. This becomes a vicious circle of negativity.

It was important to break this circle and get some positivity back into Ali's life and to create positivity circle. The basic premise to the book *The Power* by Rhonda Byrne, which is the follow up to the incredibly successful *The Secret*, is that in order for your life to truly move forward, your positive thoughts must outnumber the negative.

With the above in mind, we spent the majority of this session outlining the positive steps that she had already taken, and looked forward to the good things that would lie ahead.

Although it sometimes may seem that there is nothing to be positive about, if you look hard enough you will always find something. By finding that one thing, it is possible to reframe your current position.

For Ali, it was a case of reminding her how far she had already come and how her eventual recovery and her own personal journey could be an absolute inspiration to others.

With the above in mind I decided to use a NLP technique called Time Line Future Pacing. For this we used visualisation.

The Rules Of Visualisation

First of all I asked Ali to visualise her goal. I wanted the visualisation to be as real as possible and therefore asked her to picture the ideal scenario and describe this in as much detail as possible: what she saw, heard and felt by asking the following the questions:

See
Are you in the picture, looking at everything through your own eyes, or are you disassociated and looking at yourself as if you were a third person?
What is the location of the picture?
Is the picture in black and white or is it in colour?
Is the picture moving or is it still?
How bright are the colours in the picture?
How clear is the picture? Is everything in focus or is it blurry?
Who else is in the picture? Describe what they look like and where they are they situated.

Hear

What can you hear?

From where is the noise coming from?

Is the noise loud or soft?

Is the tone low or high? Is it soft or harsh?

How clear is the sound?

Feel

Note any inner feelings that you have.

Where is the feeling located within your body?

What shape is the feeling?

Is the feeling hard or soft?

Does this feeling move or is it static?

What is the temperature of this feeling?

Does it have a colour?

The more attention you pay to the above, the greater the visualization and the more the subconscious will have to work with.

General Guidelines about Goal Setting

Be meaningful and measureable – if your goal, for example, is to weigh less, you should state it in a way that could be measured by both you and anyone else. "I will weigh 140 pounds" is more powerful than "I will lose 10 pounds" or worse still "I will lose weight"'

Without meaningfulness and measurability, your goal is just a "want" and as such, is much less powerful.

Express the goal in the present tense – I am rather than I will

Attach an emotion to your goal and make it as powerful as possible – in Ali's case she used the expression "awesome" which can be incredibly powerful.

Always express your goal in a positive manner as your brain doesn't accept negatives. Try this and see what happens - Don't think of a pink spotted elephant.

Be specific – The more specific, the better: "I will weigh 140 pounds at 6.00pm on 24th December" is a lot more powerful than "I will weigh 140 pounds".

Write it down – when a goal is written down it will give an indication to your subconscious mind of the area in which to work. We then look to the law of attraction to provide the materials to help attract the tools to help achieve the goal. Read it as many times as possible during the day. Use dead time such as when you are waiting in a queue or stuck in traffic, as well as the beginning and the end of the day. This will help reaffirm to your subconscious exactly what is required.

This is the time when you really must be prepared to get out of your comfort zone because in order to really achieve something, you will have to learn some new skills and smash through those mental blocks that are currently holding you back.

You may wish to chunk your goal down into smaller manageable short term ones. So if the goal is, for example, to drop from 170 pounds to 140 pounds, an initial mini goal of 165 pounds for example, could be set then 160 pounds and so on until the overall goal is achieved. The main benefits of chunking down are as follows:

An initial smaller target will appear to be more easily achievable and can provide a greater incentive for you to get going. Once you have started to achieve the smaller goals, your mindset will change, and you will begin to see yourself as someone who is an achiever. This sense of achievement will become habit forming.

Once the visualisation had been set up, I made Ali walk along an imaginary timeline which started at the present day and ending at the visualisation date. Along the way she would stop at any noticeable dates which may present challenges (normally these include birthdays, weekends away etc) which may knock Ali off course. We then discussed how she would deal with the challenges in order to keep her on course.

I also encouraged Ali to stop whenever something relevant came into her head which would help her achieve her goal. Once she had reached her goal date, I asked her to turn round, look back to now and collect up all her learnings, gather them into a ball as if they were connected by string and then throw them back to now. I then asked her to walk back to the present and catch the ball and take it into her heart. Looking at this exercise from a conscious viewpoint it wouldn't seem to work, but it does. Sometimes you just have to trust your subconscious!

10: Roller coaster

2nd July 2010

It's been four weeks since I saw the consultant and guess what? I have heard nothing from the hospital. Surprise! Surprise! I have been on this roller coaster for ten months now and I have got no further with a diagnosis, a cure or a reason. So I will be interested in this visit as, unless they have been abducted by aliens, they are seriously running out of excuses. I have absolutely no faith in this hospital and realise that, as I have no money for private medicine, the cure is going to be down to me.

I have managed to feel fairly well over the last few weeks. Mum and Dad's stay was good and I enjoyed it. I was able to walk around and cook a meal. My back was giving out towards the end and I was exhausted but I left Mum and Dad feeling confident I was on the mend.

I really didn't want Mum going home depressed like last time.

My personnel manager at Tesco is still waiting to hear from my consultant, she first asked for a report at the beginning of February. When I next go to see my consultant I am going to take Suzanne with me. She has been busy lately as she and Luke got custody of Alicia. It has been a very difficult time as Alicia who is now almost three years old has been very hard work. She is clearly traumatised at being moved away from her foster mother and has reverted back to nappies. Suzanne and Luke are reassuring her all the time that she is safe and loved. Poor little munchkin has been through so much in her short life.

Suzanne is furious about the whole process I have had to go through with this illness. I am an emotional wreck when I go to see the consultant and usually end up sobbing and not asking the right questions. She is going to ask the questions that need to be asked for me. It's funny, when she was ill I was the one asking the questions because she found it so difficult. Why do we find it so hard to talk about our own health with medical professionals? It's great having kids that can sort you out in times like this. Katie has just dealt with a law firm who were trying to bill me and with hold my marriage license after I had asked them to proceed with my divorce. We had discussed legal aid and I had assumed this was how I was going to proceed as I would not be able to afford it otherwise.

Unfortunately I was so ill at the beginning of the year that I had to cancel a lot of appointments. The solicitor's office is down a cobbled street that is quite steep, there is no parking nearby and the walk there is very difficult for me. The solicitor sent out a letter to my husband and then promptly billed me £500 for it. I ignored it knowing it was a mistake but when I finally got to see him he told me I would have to pay or they would keep my marriage certificate. It is an American certificate so it is not easy to get a copy of. I got very upset and told him that I was covered by legal aid. He said that as I hadn't signed the forms yet this was not the case. I felt so helpless and vulnerable, I ended up getting very tearful and this frustrated me as I can normally deal with situations like this without a problem.

He was so arrogant and totally ignored my distress, he told me they accepted Switch, which made me feel utterly degraded as I had just told him I could not afford these legal fees while I was off sick. I left very upset and phoned Katie, my daughter who is also a solicitor. I had not asked her to sort out my divorce as I did not want her to be in the middle of anything with her father. She was livid when I told her what happened and, God bless her, she went straight into solicitor mode. She sent me a document that I had to sign that gave her the right to act on my behalf and, after telling her all the details, I left it to her. Needless to say I now have my marriage certificate and no legal bill. I have always been so tough, and normally could have dealt with that myself, but I feel so low and unable to cope with these things without getting emotional.

This is what is so disturbing about this illness. It takes away your ability to cope with the simplest of tasks. Everything you do seems such an effort, even going to the post office or the bank can exhaust you for the whole day. I do not have a disabled sticker so unless I am feeling well I do not attempt trips out. I have made it to the bank before, then have found myself unable to make it back to the car. I had to sit on a bench in the rain, until I managed to get my head around taking each step back to the car park. It was really frightening, so I am very careful now, and never go anywhere alone.

11: Dreams

13th July 2010

I saw a great saying today, so I wrote it down as it rang true with me.

'LIFE HAS PRESENTED ME WITH A BILL, AND I AM FINDING IT HARD TO PAY'.

I have a two re-occurring dreams: In the first I am in a jumbo jet cockpit with the pilot. The plane takes off but cannot get altitude and is flying too low. We are flying through a city and the pilot is dodging the sky scrapers, flying under bridges and just missing cables and the tops of buildings. My heart is in my mouth and although we never hit anything, we come so close that I am terrified. We never manage to get any higher and I always wake up.

In the second dream I am inside a house, and out the window there are tornados coming from every direction. I have children with me and I am trying to find safe places to hide them. The tornados come in all sizes and one can just pop up in the middle of a street I am running down. The big ones are terrifying, everything goes really dark and I can hear the roar. Again I wake up very disturbed.

This week I have had these dreams and I feel dreadful. There is no reason for this I can think of, but the pain has been very unpleasant. My legs especially are very sore and I have had real trouble walking. I have to sleep in shifts three hours at a time. I cannot lie for any longer as it is so uncomfortable. I am trying to be positive, but I have not had a session with Mark for a while, and I am forgetting what I should do. My head is so thick and fuzzy and I feel hungry all the time.

I have to snap out of it, I was doing so well. Can't write any more.

12: Positive

23rd July 2010

I got hold of a book today called 'The EFT Manual' by an author called Gary Craig.(energy psychology press 2008) He describes EFT as a "tool for the people helping tool box" (pg 38). That to me was a brilliant description, as in therapy I think it would be a wonderful 'tool' to use in some cases, especially for those cannot get past a difficult experience that changed their perspective on life.

I am still a little sceptical about how easy it seems, especially after all my years of study as a counsellor, but the proof is in the pudding and I am definitely the pudding! (well definitely pudding shaped!) I feel like my eyes have been opened and although I am still suffering with pain, it's manageable, it's not keeping me in bed all day. Now all I have to do is find my wings!

I have a plan now and it doesn't involve lying in bed feeling too ill to cope with life. I am coming back to health and this time it's for good. Just you wait and see!

13: Negative

27th July 2010

Mark has been on holiday for two weeks now. I have been dieting now for six weeks and have managed to lose 5lbs. I have not really had my heart in it and I cannot exercise at all because of the pain, and even though I eat healthy food, I eat too much!

You know no one wants me as a patient. I can see the defeat in their eyes when I walk in. They have no answers.

I'm sorry I am sounding a bit flat just now. I have been hurting a lot these last few days and I am hardly moving out my chair. I am trying to find positive things to look forward to, maybe it's the weather. It has been raining for days. I am scared I am going to get addicted to my pain killers, so I am trying to reduce them. They do not get rid of the pain, but they sure do take the edge off.

I am going to stop writing because this is all so depressing.

14: Doctors, consultants, medical examiners?

3rd August 2010

I went to see the consultant to day, I took Suzanne with me and we arrived to find my consultant was off sick and I was going to see her registrar. Suzanne was not happy, but in all honesty I felt I could connect with him better than with the consultant.

I had received a letter yesterday saying that I clearly had a myalgic illness and it was beyond their specialist care, which meant that their department does not deal with my sort of illness or chronic pain.

The registrar asked me about the pain and where it was. I got quite tearful because it's at these times I realise how disabled I am. Suzanne then took over and pointed out that I had come to my GP initially about 18 months ago with pain in my legs and exhaustion, not high blood pressure. The high blood pressure was a result of being put on steroids and once weaned off them the pain returned. No one has yet helped me with the pain and how tired I get. It has been nine months since I first saw the consultant and nothing has happened that can help my condition in any way.

The registrar seemed very sincere when he agreed that something needed to be done. He explained that their hands were tied about the length of time things took due to waiting lists, but he felt I had to see someone about the pain as a priority. He told us he would write to my GP with urgency and also contact the rheumatologist.

I left feeling much more confident than I usually do leaving the consultant and I feel that he really is going to help me.

I came home to a phone call from the benefits office. They were sending me to see a medical examiner - to see if I really am ill I suppose. I hate this, I almost feel a fraud already. How am I supposed to convince this person that I am ill, when my doctors don't know what is wrong with me?

Mark was back from his holiday and I needed to see him, I seem to be losing confidence in everything. I am suffering a lot of pain and have no energy. I am worrying about my forthcoming trip to Edinburgh and how I will cope.

So Mark came and I told him how sore my right leg was; it was really playing me up. He got me to concentrate and start tapping, focusing on the pain in my leg. I described it as a red, angry pain and followed his lead. Within two minutes the pain had almost gone. I was speechless. It is absolutely amazing how this works, I just wish it would work for all of my body at once.

Just talking to Mark helped me focus and I was right back on track with the self healing.

Mark's Perspective:

It is easy sometimes to get carried away with what is happening in the 'real world' and to forget the basics. As a practitioner, for the greater part of sessions I tend to use Matrix Reimprinting as I feel it cannot only remove negative emotions, beliefs and habits, but also replace them with positive ones.

However, it is important on certain occasions to get back to the basics and this is what we did on this particular occasion, Whilst talking with Ali about the current pain she was suffering it seemed apparent that it was as a result of anger that she had experienced whilst I was away and that this anger had engulfed her thinking.

What was required at this stage was to reduce the pain, and at the same time remind Ali of the power of EFT which she could then use on herself in the future. All we did at this stage was to go through the standard EFT procedure which reduced the pain. Having helped the short term problem, it was hoped that the EFT tapping would provoke more memories over the following week.

15: Progress

16th August 2010

It was great seeing everyone in Scotland. There were so many of us all visiting at once, it was a great family get together. I was lucky enough to be staying with Aunt Kathryn, so had huge double bed to myself. I slept really well and the pain certainly subsided. However I found I got extremely tired when we were all together. There were so many people and children, all talking at once. I managed to get time to myself and continued tapping. My arms, shoulders and neck had gone very stiff probably because of the long drive, so I would work on them when I lay in bed.

I had long talks with Aunt Kathryn about things that I remembered from my childhood and it was rather good to learn about my memories from someone else's perspective. You see things so differently when you are a child.

I also got together with Fran, my cousin's wife's sister, who had suffered from ME and fibromyalgia for five years. Like me it took a long time getting diagnosed and she thought she was losing her mind. In fact one doctor told her that she was at the doctors way too much for someone in their 20's, and he would put it down to the fact that she was Italian.

Fran was mortified and, already down because of the illness, was losing all hope of ever getting better or even being diagnosed. Like me she also scanned the internet and got confused with all the possibilities that were out there. She finally got taken seriously and was sent for some trials for ME sufferers, where she was given Cognitive Behavioural Therapy treatment and also saw a specialist in unusual diseases. Neither of these helped particularly, but during the trials she did get to meet other sufferers.

One thing that became apparent was that it was not lazy people who got this illness, in fact the majority of people work in full time jobs, run businesses and are always on the go. This brings me back to my point at the beginning regarding recognising the symptoms before it's too late.

Fran also met another lady who had had ME for six years, recovered and then got breast cancer, which thankfully she also recovered from. She told Fran that breast cancer was easier to cope with compared to how she felt with ME. As Fran progressed through her illness she was told about something called 'Leaky Gut Syndrome' which is a condition caused by a damaged bowel lining.

This can occur due to toxins, poor diet or medications to name a few. With fibromyalgia and ME you find irritable bowel syndrome becomes part and parcel of it. In my case it was the least of my worries as I have suffered from that for many years, just as I had accepted depression as a way of life, I never once suspected it had anything to do with my illness. However many alternative practitioners believe it is the start of other problems such as Rheumatoid Arthritis, Crohn's disease, Lupus, Fibromyalgia, MS and Chronic Fatigue syndrome (ME).

The treatment for this condition is a gluten and casein free diet. This involves eating no wheat or dairy products.

So Fran tried it. It took a little while but gradually things began to improve. First to disappear was her fibromyalgia, which meant she was pain free. The tiredness took longer to heal but gradually over time it did. She is married now with a baby and has learnt how to pace herself. She knows if she over does things she may have a bad day, so she will have that cup of tea after doing the vacuuming instead of rushing onto the next job.

It was very therapeutic talking to her; it is always good to know that you are not the only one out there. It seems so strange to me that we all seem to suffer from the same ailments, so why is it so difficult for our doctors to diagnose and treat? I have decided to try the gluten and dairy free diet. If anything it may help me lose weight, but if it does help with the pain then that will be a bonus.

16: DWP Medical Assessment

17th August 2010

I know I only wrote yesterday, but I have to tell you about this. I went for a medical assessment today arranged by the benefits office as I have just started to claim Employment and Support Allowance. I guess they want to see if I am faking it or am actually unfit for work.

I know there is lots of pressure on at the moment with the new government wanting to get people back to work, so I was a little apprehensive and unsure what to expect.

The doctor was an older gentleman who seemed very pleasant. I started to explain everything that happened but he cut me off, saying that he was only here to find out how this illness is affecting me. He asked me a series of questions and then spent a lot of time typing in the computer. He again seemed to focus on my high blood pressure and depression, even though I tried to explain that the tiredness and the pain were having a much worse affect on my day to day living. He asked how I had travelled to the clinic and if anyone had come with me. I told him I had driven myself and parked close by.

He then asked if I watched TV; I told him I did. He then asked me what I watched. I was a little confused but I answered him, telling him I liked the documentaries and sci fi programmes

He continued to type into the computer and I was none the wiser.

He asked if I could read a book or sit at a computer, all of which I answered yes to. I tried to tell him that all these things I do when I am well enough to do them, but I guess there was no tick box for that on his computer. I also told him I studied a lot, but I don't know if I should have volunteered that.

He asked how many shirts I could iron at once; I said two before I had to sit down. He then got me to bend my legs a little, took my blood pressure (which was fine), tapped me with his hammer to see my reflexes and poked me in the back (which bloody hurt). None of these things were particularly stressful, but I wondered if they should be.

Does this mean they are going to say I am fit for work? I don't know what I will do if that is the case. I clearly cannot do any active work and I am not sure how I will cope with a desk job, if I can get one, I certainly couldn't do a full day. Some days I would not be able to go in at all and who would employ me with this medical record. Maybe I am worrying too much.

I have to wait four weeks for the report and diagnosis which apparently is computer generated from what information the doctor has put in. This is incredible, the computer is going to tell me what is wrong? If I had known that I would just have asked my computer instead of wasting the time of all these consultants!

17: A series of positive events

27th August 2010

Well this week has been a series of positive events. Firstly I passed my advanced diploma in counselling, which was a major relief after all the classes I missed due to this illness. I am now qualified.

I also went into work and spoke to my Personnel Manager who is applying for me to be retired on ill health grounds; this means I could have access to the pension I have paid, which isn't much but it will help.

I also got a call from the NHS long term illness support group and have been put on a six week course starting in October to help me cope with being ill, and then finally, and almost best of all, I went to the doctors and saw a young female doctor I have not seen before. The registrar I saw on the 3rd of August did do what he had promised, he wrote to my GP and recommended that I get seen by an ME specialist and so the ball is now rolling and the young doctor was happy to put me forward and finally diagnose me.

In one respect I am relieved that I am finally going to get some help with this, but on the other hand, I have to question the amount of time this has taken and the amount of pain I have endured without reason or cause.

The gluten and dairy free diet did nothing to either change my symptoms nor my weight and after three weeks I gave up. It was so difficult and expensive as the gluten free products are very over priced. If it had been a miracle cure then I would have gone on, but nothing changed at all, except for the colour of my stools!

However it definitely worked for Fran, so it may be that for some people it will help. I would certainly recommend you try it, so you can at least rule it out if it doesn't. I'm afraid with this condition you have to get used to being your own doctor. Yesterday the kids were round, I love seeing them but I cannot cope with them for long as I get too exhausted and sore. I look at these babies and think about what they have both been through in their very short lives; Skye who was born at 26 weeks weighing 1lb 10oz, is like a little spider monkey now. She is not yet walking but can get anywhere at the speed of light, you cannot take your eyes off her for a second. She is still tiny, but smiles all the time and has a massive attitude; she has no fear whatsoever and yells at you in a very loud voice if you are not taking notice of her. The other day she was strapped into her high chair and Alicia was eating at the table. Suzanne popped to the loo and when she came back Skye had wriggled out of her straps and had climbed onto the table and was sitting there eating Alicia's leftovers.

Alicia is now settled with Suzanne and Luke as her mummy and daddy. It has been difficult, the poor toddler was so confused. It did not help that Maxine insisted that Alicia call her mummy during her supervised visits and got angry with her when she didn't. Social Services had to intervene and every time Alicia saw Max a rash would appear on her face and she would have terrible tantrums during the course of the following few days. She has now not seen her for six weeks and is in a secure loving routine with Suzanne and Luke, who would love to adopt her as their own. She is such a happy little thing and I wish it could all be sorted.

Unfortunately Maxine is still pulling the strings whenever she can. We guessed she was pregnant again and Suzanne pulled her aside and asked her. She admitted that she was and said that Social Services had known since the court case back in May. Suzanne was furious as no one had bothered to tell her and., as she was the carer for Alicia she was worried how this would affect the child if Max suddenly showed up with another baby. Also, was Maxine going to be allowed to keep this baby? No one seemed to know. How were we supposed to explain this to Alicia? Maxine behaves like she has been the world's best mother and if you didn't know her you would almost believe it. The fact that she never actually asks how Alicia is coping or seems to care about her feelings are completely missing in this strange behaviour. She talks like and treats Alicia like her possession and expects things of her that are way too advanced for a child of three. She also assumes that Alicia misses her and asks for her. She seems to have completely forgotten that she only had Alicia for a few months and in that time she neglected her terribly. She then only saw Alicia a couple of times a week for supervised visits so Alicia does not miss her at all, but Max just refuses to understand this. The truth is that Alicia only asks about her foster mother Lynn, who still sees her every week as Suzanne meets up with her regularly. Lynn has been fantastic; she and her husband had Alicia for almost three years, on and off, love her dearly and would have adopted her if she had not gone to Suzanne. Alicia loves them very much and Suzanne makes sure they maintain a regular relationship. This has helped Alicia settle in, but not once has she asked for Maxine.

Maxine will not allow Suzanne to adopt her, even though she is about to have another baby with yet another boyfriend. It is so unfair when you think that poor Suzanne has struggled so much trying to help her.

I also hope that once this child is born in November that she starts to leave Suzanne alone. She is allowed a visit with Alicia in September, but only under the condition that she does not refer to herself as mummy or to the new baby as a sibling,so, as you can see, I still have loads on my plate.

You would never believe the text message I have just received off my ex-husband. He is sitting in a pub and has just text me to ask if I would look after the kids so Suzanne and Robyn can go round to paint his house for him. I did not reply even though I could think of lots of expletives I could have used. I was actually toying with the idea of asking him for some money to help me support his children as I am not working now, but I guess The Queens Arms needs it more than they do.

I must be feeling good as I am still sitting here typing, so if you still feel like reading I must fill you in on my last visit from Mark.

I have been in a lot of pain since my holiday in Edinburgh especially my arms, wrists and hands. I think that is probably from holding the steering wheel on that long drive. It has been getting me down a bit, but I had to prepare for a group of psychodynamic counsellors coming over for an evening to discuss EFT/Matrix reimprinting with Mark.

There were 13 of us in total and it was a very fascinating night. Poor Mark was bombarded with lots of scientific facts and I realised that a lot of the group were quite sceptical. It was very interesting to see how he handled the group and then demonstrated some of the techniques he uses. They were very impressed and interested in how it could work for them. As I become more aware of how the Matrix works I can actually see the benefits of combining both skills. Using our counselling skills we can work with clients and help them discover the reasons behind their thought processes and behaviours. It can be a difficult journey for the client while they uncover difficult memories that have been buried a long time and this can sometimes leave them feeling bewildered and empty. Using Matrix Reimprinting you could then help the client make the memories easier to remember and then move on from them.

Mark came round on the Friday afterwards and helped me with pain relief. It did help a bit but not enough to get me through the day. I'm afraid I still am reliant on a lot of pain killers.

We then decided to work on a memory that I found difficult. I went back to another birthday I'd had, where my ex came home very drunk and very mean. He staggered in the door and threw some garage flowers at me as the girls had called him and reminded him it was my birthday. I ignored him and he grabbed a drink and went to lie on the sofa to watch his new 42" plasma TV screen that we couldn't afford. He couldn't get any volume and he went crazy, throwing things around and screaming at the kids blaming them. He was very angry and scary; the kids ran upstairs and I decided to take them out to the cinema. All the time Craig was telling me that the volume was just turned down. We all got in the car and he came out and stood in front of the car screaming at me. I was humiliated because of my neighbours, and scared and upset.

So Mark took me back into this memory tapping on me; I pictured myself in the car with the kids in the back. Mark told me to take myself into the picture with my ECHO and tap on myself driving the car. I could see myself sitting next to me in the front of the car. He asked me what I wanted to do, I said I wanted to run him over. Mark said "Do it then".

So in my mind I put the car into gear and drove forward. I then realised the kids were in the back of the car and they would get upset if I ran over their dad, no matter how horrible he was, so instead I just drove forward until I had pinned him up against the garage door and he couldn't move. I stared at him with this 'Will I? Won't I?' look until I saw fear in his eyes, I then laughed at him and so did the kids. I felt so much better about that horrible day then and now I see him pinned against the garage door when I think of it.

Mark's Perspective:

The lesson from this session I think is that once the memory is reimprinted, it stays that way (unless of course you reimprint the reimprintment!) Every time Ali tries to remember that particular memory, all she sees is the fear in the eyes of a person who previously had put fear into her. This was another "bad tree in the forest of memories " that had been chopped down and replaced by a new, good tree. We were getting closer to the point where the good trees were going to outnumber the bad trees and that place where Rhonda Byrne believes we can all move forward.

18: Autumn now approaching

17th September 2010

Gosh! It has been a while and there is so much to say; everything seems to be so tough at the moment, but I am refusing to be beaten. I am not sure where to start, I have gone back to my journal to remind me of the last few weeks and it is not comfortable reading.

I received a letter from the DWP to tell me that my Employment and Support Allowance had been stopped as the computer generated medical report had deemed me fit to work. I was allowed to appeal and so I did, this means that the money will be reinstated until I attend a hearing at a later date. I am not surprised but find it totally ridiculous as none of the questions I was asked related to my illness in anyway. Katie came home for a week and was extremely uptight and stressed; she was biting everyone's head off. I tried to talk to Katie over dinner one night, but it resulted in tears almost from the start. She is so fragile at the moment, she just spends her whole life working and seems to forgotten how to have fun. She is so tired, which makes her very defensive and that in itself can manifest into hostility if you push her too far.

I was so worried after Katie went home I didn't sleep for three nights, tossing and turning, wondering what I could do to help her. Of course worry, along with every other negative emotion, triggers the symptoms and before long the exhaustion was overwhelming and the pain in my back unbearable. I was trying to grab sleep at intervals and having horrible dreams, one in particular was driving into flood water with Katie in the car and trying to get out.

When Mark came round I was so shattered that he decided to use EFT to take me on a journey to my future self.

First we made a list of things I want :

I will be an excellent counsellor, I will start a new job, I will be pain free and 100% better, I will be healthy and content with myself, Suzanne will be completely better, I will be earning enough money to be more supportive to my kids, I will be helping people cope with ME, Katie will have gone travelling, Suzanne will be able to adopt Alicia, I will get a dog again and go for long walks feeling fit and happy.

Then while Mark tapped on me I imagined myself a year from now: I was walking along the canal with a new crazy dog jumping up at me and chasing the ducks. It was a warm windy day and I was invigorated, confident and happy. As I walked I came across myself (as I am now) sitting on a bench by a bridge. I looked tired and ill. So I sat next to the present me and started to explain about my journey over the upcoming year. I achieved nearly everything on my list and am moving forward all the time. Everyone is happy and healthy and the world is a new and exciting place for me. I am no longer in any pain and am able to lose weight with diet and exercise.

As Mark tapped I could focus very clearly on what was being said and I felt enlightened. I sent that vision out to the universe and felt so much better. When I drive through the village I see people going out walking with their dogs and I really wish I could be doing that again. I miss it so much so it was really significant for me that I saw myself walking with my dog. When Mark had gone I felt very calm and started to focus on what lay ahead. Money is a real obstacle for me right now, but so far I am managing to pay everything. With Craig starting college I have to add another £50 a week travel costs. We will have to cut back so Sky TV is going along with my beloved cans of diet coke. Sounds crazy, but we get through loads in this family, real diet coke addicts, it cost a small fortune!

Mark's Perspective:

This session used a technique called Matrix Future Reimprinting which owes a fair bit to the Time Line NLP process that we had used previously.

It relies on having a clear picture of who and where you want to be in the future and using your future ECHO to guide you to that place. The whole debate of whether the past and future actually exist could be brought in at this point, but as the point of this book is tell a story of recovery, I think that the debate is best left to persons far more intellectual than I am! Matrix Future Reimprinting seems somehow to be more powerful than straightforward visualisation. Maybe it is because we are literally tapping into our own subconscious and telling it what we want to attract into our lives.

19: Maxine

25th September 2010

I think it's about time I explained Maxine's story to you. You see people don't understand the difference of having a teenager going off the rails and having someone like Maxine. I feel such anger towards her just now and anger is not a healthy emotion.

I think in all honesty when it was me she was hurting directly I could cope more, but now it is Suzanne and Alicia that she is affecting I am seeing red.

I always knew there was something not completely right with her from the beginning, she was very destructive with possessions and had constant tantrums. I made allowances as I was in no doubt that these children had had a terrible time. Maxine had been totally neglected, with only her older sisters there to take care of her and they were only young children themselves.

By the time she was seven and I was pregnant with Craig, it was becoming a real problem. The school was beginning to lose patience with her strange behaviour, she told the most outrageous lies and was always disruptive, for example, she got rid of her shoes one day and told her teacher that we couldn't afford shoes. I'd take her to school in the mornings and stay until the bell rang, watch her go in and then get a phone call a couple of hours later to say she hadn't appeared. She would be hiding in the open plan buildings, making children laugh by poking her head up every now and then. They were all childish pranks, albeit scary for someone so young to be doing. The worst thing for me was the look on her face when she behaved badly. She would always do the opposite of what you said and then stare at you with these blank eyes waiting for your reaction, almost as if she wasn't there. One time in particular was on a trip to Scotland to visit my Aunt Kathryn who had recently lost her beloved dog. my aunt was very upset by it and I told the kids not to mention the dog unless she did. We all walked into the house and the first thing Max did was ask where the dog was, all the time staring at me straight in the eyes waiting for my reaction.

I began to feel like I was going mad. Here was a young child who surely could not be that manipulative. I over compensated, taking her on special days out, making her birthdays huge and exciting, but it never changed. At Christmas there always used to be loads of gifts for everyone. Max would open her gifts expressionless and be watching what all the other kids got, it somehow always ended up her taking their toys and frequently breaking them. I took her to see a children's counsellor but it proved to be pointless. I am sure Maxine manipulated everything that was said and acted the part brilliantly; she was in control the whole time. When she was nine her class was taken to a music festival performance at Buxton Opera House, I was reluctant to let her go as I did not trust her at all by then, But her teacher phoned me and promised me she would keep an eye on her if I allowed her to go, so I gave in. I picked her up from the school later and she behaved as if everything was fine. When I got in the same teacher phoned me to say I had been right and she should have listened. Max had snuck away at an interval and then proceeded to have what looked like a full blown epileptic fit in the foyer. They called an ambulance and when the teacher found her she was lying on the floor, surrounded by concerned officials. The teacher (who was also wise to her by this stage), told her to get up at once. Maxine stood up absolutely fine with a smirk on her face. That was her last ever trip.

By the time she was 11, she was also a bully. I had many parents complain about her but none stand out more than the distressed woman who banged on my door absolutely furious because Max had been bullying her daughter at the park, she had then phoned the mother and told her a strange man had pulled up and taken her daughter away. The woman was frantic and Max just stood smirking whilst I apologised profusely. Punishments were hard. They were in fact a waste of time, also her father did not back me up. He worked away all week and drank at the pub all weekend so never had to deal with parents, teachers and her behaviour.

When Maxine started high school, her hormones kicked in and all hell broke loose. The school was on the phone almost daily as her behaviour was horrendous. She bullied teachers and students alike. She was violent and started drinking and taking drugs. Her behaviour was also outrageous; I caught her urinating in the drain outside our house one day and she also started a fire in the woods and burnt Craig's hand in it.

She had a gang of kids, who were all younger than her, follow her around everywhere. Lots of other parents would not let their children near her, it was so humiliating, I just didn't know what to do and no one would help me.

She started skipping school, but when she was caught and suspended she then insisted on being in school and would sneak in any way she could. I tried to get her part time jobs, but she was sacked almost immediately. I don't know what she told people about me but I felt like eyes were on me all the time, even going to the local shops. I had to have a hysterectomy and, whilst I was recovering in bed, Maxine went to some friend's house and told them I had gone to Scotland with all the family and locked her out the house so she had to sleep on the streets. When she didn't come home for the night I phoned the police who found her surrounded by all her friends the next day. This would be a regular occurrence and the police were visitors at my house at least twice a week. Every time they caught her, she would get violent and attack them. There was not much they could do as she was only 14, so they would just bring her back screaming and kicking. One morning I came down the stairs and found my phone was dead. I later found out Max had cut the wire as she had been suspended again and did not want me to get the phone call. It didn't work as the educational officer came to our house. She had been suspended this time as she had terrorised a young girl in the toilets at school. Apparently they had never seen anything quite like this attack and the girl's father was after her blood; he wanted the police involved.

All this was bad, but the worst was yet to come. By now Suzanne and Katie had both gone to university so Maxine decided she could come and go as she pleased and ignored all the house rules. The trouble was she was drunk all the time and coming in at anytime she wanted. I couldn't stop her and she was wrecking the house; she was peeing on the floor of her room, dropping plates of food when she staggered about and would strip naked all the time, she also completely blanked out and did not know anything she was doing. One night she terrified Craig by going into his room naked and very drunk and screaming at the top of her head. I had to manhandle her out to her room. I couldn't sleep at all, as I lay listening out for her so I could protect the other kids when she came in. Eventually I locked the doors and left the garage door open. She came back and I told her that unless she obeyed the house rules she would not get back in. She was 15 and I was at the end of my tether. I called Social Services but they were not interested. I went to the doctorasking for psychological help for her but he just laughed at me and said that he couldn't do that for every parent that was having trouble with their teenager.

Maxine lived in the garage for about three months. She had been expelled from school by then and was drinking all the time. Every now and then I would get her in and we would talk, she would cry and say that she wanted to change and I would say I wanted to help her. It wouldn't last a day; she would go back out the minute my back was turned. The last of these occasions was the turning point for me. She had been in the house promising that she was now ready to get help; she had a shower and some dinner and then disappeared. At 9.30pm I got a phone call from the police cells. All I could hear was roaring and banging in the background, it sounded like a wild animal going beserk in its cage.

The policeman who rang told me that they had arrested Max because she was ramming shopping trolleys into the sides of cars in Tesco's car park. He said he had never seen anything like this in his 25 years on the force. She was incredibly violent and the noise I could hear was her attacking the door of the cell. He said I could get her in the morning but she was not safe to be let out that night. I started to cry and I told him I really didn't want to get her ever. He said he would ring Social Services. I told him I had already phoned them but they would not help me. He said that they had to help me if I refused to have her back. So that was what I did, I refused, and when Social Services came round, even the guilt trip they tried to place on me could not even touch the humiliation and shame I had felt over the last few years trying to make excuses for her behaviour. I had been utterly helpless and they had not offered me any help so I did not feel guilty, the only thing I felt was relief. So she went into a foster home and they thought she was wonderful. Of course that grated on my nerves. Maxine had been brought up properly so knew how to behave well and speak properly but she only turned it on when she felt like it. Of course it didn't last. She suddenly realised her freedom was gone and that the foster home had house rules the same as every other home. She blew her top and accused the foster father of trying to sexually molest her. This wasn't a new thing for Maxine, she had already tried to accuse her father and a teacher of that in the past. So she became un-fosterable and was, at the age of 16, given her own flat. This started a new era where she could pretty much do what she liked and was given money to do it. She destroyed the flat; it was disgusting, so they gave her another one. Meantime her criminal record was growing and she was well known for being hard and violent. People were scared of her it seemed, everyone except her family. She had hooked up with another delinquent, and they spent most of the time beating each other up. She was always injured and covered in bruises. I tried every now and then to help her when she was really broken. She would move home, be great for a couple of weeks then it would all start again and she would move back in with this lad.

During all these years Biff was no support to me at all. He just didn't want to know and didn't want her in the house. He worked down in Exeter all week and spent every weekend in the pub. We rowed all the time but he was always too drunk to be rational. This was not helping the other kids in the house, let alone Maxine.

Over the next five years I think she ruined every Christmas and it got to a point where none of us had anything to do with her.

She kept getting pets, dogs mainly, but she would mistreat them. They never got toilet trained so they defecated all over her stuff. We managed to re-home a lot of animals taken from her and we kept one little dog that had been so poorly treated with all its teeth kicked out of its head. I doubt that she would have done that as she loves animals, but her drunken boyfriend was a prime candidate. When she was 20 she had been badly beaten by her boyfriend and I let her move home again. Suzanne offered to let her live with her in London.

I sometimes thought that neither Suzanne nor Katie really appreciated how dreadful she had become as they were away at university during these last few years. She did not last long in London. She almost destroyed Suzanne's home, physically attacked her friends and was what they could only describe as psychotic. I remember Luke admitting to me that he could not believe Maxine was as bad as I had described until he lived with her. He hadn't read or seen anything like this in all his years of journalism. His words in his Irish accent were "She is completely mental!"

Her personal hygiene was always a serious problem. She refused to brush her teeth. She rarely washed and would put makeup on top of old makeup. She smelt of stale alcohol and it was making their shared home stink. Suzanne tried to talk to her as I had done but the situation just got worse. In the end Suzanne frog marched Max back to Macclesfield after she had smashed all the dishes in their house and taken a bite out of one of their flat mate's arms while he had tried to restrain her. He had had to go to hospital and she had locked herself in a room - they virtually had to break the door down to get her out. They got off the train in Macclesfield and Max disappeared again for a while, although we heard terrible stories of her exploits every now and then.

That was until she re-appeared at the age of 21, six months pregnant with Alicia. She was still drinking then, but told me it was just a glass a night. I guess I didn't believe her, but I wanted to believe it for the sake of the baby.

She was back with this lad she used to fight with, Alicia's father. I helped them get a rented house and helped them move from another place they had destroyed. I set up the baby's room but I don't know why I thought it would be any different. Four days after Alicia was born Maxine went to a party with her and got absolutely wasted. A stranger ended up taking Alicia home and taking care of her. Things went from bad to worse; the house they lived in was disgusting, empty bottles of vodka and wine everywhere. The landlord kept phoning me saying he was going to chuck them out. I tried to make her see sense but it was a waste on time. I went round one day and there was broken glass in the Moses' basket and blood up the wall. They had had another drunken fight. They were evicted and she was homeless, staying in all sorts of places with the baby. I couldn't find them so I rang Social Services. They had already had reports, but were also concerned. Eventually she was located and I said they could stay with me until a place at a mother baby unit was discovered. That lasted three days. She popped out for milk at 10am on the second morning and the next time I saw her was 10pm at night, absolutely out of her face on drugs and alcohol. She was demanding the baby. I gave Alicia to Robyn and then told her to get out of my house. She went for me but was so drunk that I just pushed her away and she fell over. She stood up then fell backwards down the stairs. I phoned the police and she ran away.

Alicia was taken into care a few days later. Maxine completely blacked out and did not know where she was for 48 hours. She just cried and cried, she knew it was wrong, but she just couldn't stop. When she cries you feel so sorry for her, it's heartbreaking, but she can stop crying and change personality quicker than you could blink. It's very scary to watch someone hysterical with grief one minute and then bouncing with laughter the next. So now Suzanne and Luke have fostered Alicia but Maxine still causes trouble whenever she can. She is due to have another baby soon, God help that child, because I will not get involved this time. I cannot go through anymore of the turmoil that will happen. I am still in shock that Social Services seem to be allowing this pregnancy to carry on as normal. According to Maxine everything is fine and she is allowed to keep the baby. Deep down my head is telling me not to believe her but I have not seen or heard anything to the contrary. The only positive twist to this is that the guy she has hooked up with just now seems a lot smarter than the other ones. He has a job which is a bonus and is really excited about this child. At the moment he earns good money, working nights, and gives Max whatever she wants. She is a very attractive girl when she is clean and he probably thinks he has hit the lottery. She is wearing nice clothes and jewellery, has her hair and nails done and they eat out a lot.

He also got her a dog and two cats, which I know is a recipe for disaster.

The problem I was aware of was that he was around when Alicia was getting neglected and so that leaves me feeling very worried for this new baby.

You see when the baby comes she will be unable to get into a routine; no matter how much she thinks she can do it, she won't. She feeds off drama and excitement and the mundane life of a housewife with a new baby will not fit into her world. She will not keep the house clean, get up when the baby cries nor stop her party lifestyle. I know it, Social Services know it, her sisters know it, but her poor boyfriend doesn't get it. The fact that Social Services are going to be watching this child every step of the way still has not rung alarm bells with him, but as I said she tells incredible lies and is extremely manipulative. So Maxine at the moment is kicking up a huge drama about her visitation with Alicia. She is accusing Suzanne of not telling her anything and her boyfriend is being very hostile with us.

Last Monday I took Suzanne to the cancer hospital in Manchester for a check up. She has not been great and I know she is concerned. She had a number of tests done and we have to wait for the results. She also has to have another MRI scan. The next day was a meeting with Maxine and Social Services. There were about ten people at this meeting and Maxine marched in late, made up to the nines, with an aggressive attitude. She blanked Suzanne and demanded that her boyfriend be allowed visitation with Alicia.

Of course he is not allowed visitation with a child that is not even his, but that didn't stop her and the whole meeting was a farce with Social Services trying to pacify Max and in doing so making Suzanne feel like utter shit. Suzanne phoned me to come get her and as I drove into the college gates there she was standing in the rain with her hood pulled over her head looking ill and exhausted.

I just feel so angry now. Attacking me is one thing, but attacking Suzanne and Alicia is a whole different kettle of fish. Max was a damaged child, who knows what she actually went through during the first four years of her life. The damage was already done, her personality already formed and her attachment ability was shot. I did my best but I had no idea how to deal with a damaged child. I took everything as a personal attack on me and spent years guilt ridden because I couldn't help her. It was frightening, uncontrollable and devastating and there is no doubt this also played a huge part in this illness. I spent twenty years trying to help her and it just wore me down. I don't see her at all now,. I think it is better to stay away. My body cannot handle any more stress and I just have nothing left to give. It's time to call it a day.

20: Money

3rd October 2010

I have been poorly this last week. With this condition I don't know if it's anxiety or just the condition itself. I think it's safe to say that whenever I am stressed then my symptoms definitely get worse and I think my stress levels have currently exceeded the norm.

The first subject I would like to address is Maxine again as it is playing on my mind. Writing the last chapter was therapeutic and helped me get a deeper level of understanding of everyone's emotions. I know deep down Max is very damaged and I should have more patience, however I am no angel and it is difficult. I spoke to Mark about it and we agreed hanging on to that anger was a very negative emotion and tried to work on it using EFT. The trouble was I was still angry and I don't think I wanted to let that go. It is a defense mechanism for me and I have realised the reason behind it.

Mark asked me to choose a particular moment that I wanted to change in relation to Maxine. I decided to bring back the memory of the social worker coming to me when I finally would not allow Maxine back in my house.

I had been made to feel guilty and heartless for my decision then and I wanted to change that. So Mark began tapping and I stepped into the past again. This time I sat next to my ECHO on the sofa facing the social worker. I told myself that I was doing the right thing and that I was not to feel guilty or allow these people to make me feel guilty in any way. I had asked for their help many times and had been ignored and treated like a helpless mother who couldn't handle their out of control teenager.

I felt myself getting angry and when Mark asked me if I wanted anyone else in the memory I said no, I could handle it myself.

So me and my ECHO faced this woman and told her in no uncertain terms that they had failed us as a family. They had left me to cope with a child who was seriously disturbed, and had put us all in danger of being harmed and that now it was up to them to get Maxine the psychiatric help she so desperately needed. I then sent my ECHO to get Maxine's clothes and I told the social worker that one day I would come back and tell the world how badly they had handled this. I then allowed my ECHO to give the woman the bag of clothes and we opened the door and told her to go. I then hugged my ECHO and told her that was the best thing I could have done, not only for me and the kids, but for Max also.

I think Mark was surprised at how forceful I had got but it was a good memory for me to deal with. I felt better about it immediately.

Maxine's next baby is due next month, and I am very frightened of seeing the child and getting dragged into another existence of hell where I have to watch from the sidelines whilst this child is neglected. Worse than that, is that Suzanne will have to do that as she still has to remain in touch with Max because of Alicia. I don't know how Suzanne will cope if she suspects the baby is in trouble, it is so heart breaking.

Then, out of the blue, Maxine phoned Suzanne yesterday and she could not have been nicer, which was a surprising change. She told Suzanne she had just been at court about the new baby. I cannot tell you how relieved I am. At the very least they are investigating the safety of the new baby and Maxine will be watched. Mind you, she was watched last time, but Alicia still had to go through hell before they took her. I do not feel so angry now and am so relieved for that child. I can only say what I have said a thousand times before, maybe this time she will get it together and be a good mother. Her boyfriend seems to have the makings of being a good father so only time will tell.

Mark's Perspective:

Whenever someone's ECHO shows a high level of emotion it is great, even if that emotion is anger. After all, it is negative beliefs that we are trying to eradicate and they come from negative emotions about a memory. The memory, once reimprinted, gave Ali a vehicle to offload a great deal of pent-up anger and her feelings afterwards were as a direct result of this.

This session also reiterated the important aspect of Matrix Reimprinting, which is to ensure that the ECHO is left with a positive belief rather than the negative one that had been carried around, often for a number of years. Instead of feeling guilty and heartless for her decision to not let Maxine back into her life, her ECHO, and therefore Ali, realised that the decision to leave Maxine to her own devices was best for all concerned

The next subject is money and what little of it I have. This last month has been a series of financial nightmares. First was the news of Craig's travel costs to college, quickly followed by our ancient computer breaking down. I desperately need a computer for my work and repairing it it cost me £140. My car then managed to fail its MOT and so another £200 later I was flat broke. Suzanne loaned me the £200 which I paid her back the next week from my child benefit and employment and sickness allowance. I then started my last year at uni, only to be given the devastating news that the course fees had gone up 150% to £2,500.

It might as well have been £250,000 as I just didn't have it and couldn't see how I was going to manage it. I also need £80 for the BACP membership, liability insurance and CRB checks.

I have nothing to fall back on but I have written to every student finance place I can find and am hoping something comes up. I cannot get any sort of loan due to my illness and I would not be able to pay it back anyway. Oh, and just one last thing to add on the finance front, I discovered by a sheer fluke that Biff has gone on a fly/drive holiday to Las Vegas and California with his mates. Yes the same Biff who sat in my house two weeks ago and told me that he was really sorry, he would try to help if he could, but he had no money. He actually played the role beautifully, almost had me feeling sorry for him. I had just accepted the fact he has no money and now I feel very stupid. Even now I still fall for his lies, you would think being made bankrupt as he drank and partied our house away would have woken me up but no, I'm still stupid, clearly. I'm not sure what I am going to do about this yet, but I am thinking.

I was at a workshop last Sunday learning about co-dependency. It was a long day, my back was barely holding out in these seats, but I managed to stay. One of the main revelations that came out of this lesson was my intense desire to not be dependent on anyone. After years with Biff, being the mother figure in that relationship, I have learnt the only one I can rely on is me. In some respects this may be looked upon as being strong, but in actual fact I think it's a flaw. Distrust can be harmful, and can hold you back from being in a warm loving relationship.

The thought of a relationship makes me shudder, yet this is sad, I was never like this before, when did this happen to me? When did I stop going out? When did I start hiding away from the world? I was a very attractive woman who attracted a lot attention. Now I hide under a layer of fat and baggy clothes. I feel safe, yet I am clearly not happy with how I look. I have started on a journey with Mark where I am exploring memories that were so deeply tucked away they almost did not exist anymore. As each one comes to light then so do ten more. At first I was sceptical that this would do me good but I actually do think it is working now. I am finding answers one by one.

At the moment I feel a lot better than I did. I am either getting used to the physical pain or it is improving. I still have problems walking any distance at all. I cannot make it to the butchers and back without my legs seizing up and it's only a ten minute walk there and back, yet I can manage to shop around the supermarket with a trolley. If my mind is pre occupied then I seem to get further before noticing the pain.

My legs feel so weak now I really want to find a way of exercising to firm them up again. I just don't know what to do, maybe Mark will come up with some ideas. My head is clearer today, although it has been in what I can only describe as a thick fog all week. It has been a difficult time, yet I have handled it much better, using tapping to relax myself and keep on with the affirmations.

Its been a battle, but I can see the grass beginning to grow again on the battlefield.

21: Always look to the positive

22nd October 2010

It's been a busy few weeks. Lots of positive things have happened so let me begin.

Mark had suggested I look back into negative parts of my childhood. I found it difficult to form clear memories and I sometimes think I get confused with certain situations. I looked up Sigmund Freud's psychosexual stages of development and tried to match them with my own life.

The first stage is the 'oral stage' which, in very, very brief terms, develops your trust. I was loved, cherished and protected by my parents.

During infancy and early childhood (the 'anal' and 'phallic' stages') I had to go into hospital twice for operations which were both extremely traumatising as in those days your parents could not stay with you. The latency stage followed and as I had surgery on my eyes, I had to wear glasses with a patch over the lens. We moved to Edinburgh and the kids at my new school were horrible to me and teased me all the time. I was a painfully shy child and things did not really improve for me until I finally left that school and moved down to England but the damage had already been done.

During the 'latency stage' you form relationships and learn how to socialise with school, playmates, sports and other activities.

I felt inferior and unpopular and so when I arrived at my new school in England my expectations were low, yet because of my accent I became immediately popular and I loved it.

The trouble was I would do anything to remain popular and as the 'genital stage' of development took hold, I became self destructive to impress and show off to others. I was still terrified of being alone, yet I would act tough, steal sweeties from a shop, be the first to do daring exploits and, as I got older, I smoked, drank alcohol, swore and played truant from school. I was Mum and Dad's nightmare, but of course I grew up.

I was lucky I had been loved and cared for during these early infancy stages and so began to identify more with that as I got older.

Mark felt it would be good to work on some of these situations I had had as a young child, so I picked the time when I was at school in Edinburgh, feeling lonely and scared by the other children in my class.

He began tapping on me as I went into that memory and for the first time in many years it became very real to me. I watched myself head down, with my glasses on, drawing on a piece of paper. The classroom was dark as the windows were very high up and it seemed cold and grey outside. I didn't speak or make eye contact with the other children, I didn't see the point as they would only laugh at me.

Mark told me to introduce myself as I am now to the little girl that was me. I sat down next to her and picked up a pencil and helped her draw. I told her that it was ok, that these kids were just silly and that I was an amazing person who was going to have lots of friends very soon.

She didn't look at me and I wanted to cry. Mark was still tapping so he asked me to bring someone else in that may help so I brought my gran into the scene. The other kids could not see her so she was being naughty; she went and stuck her tongue out at the mean girl and flicked her pen out her hand. Little Alison giggled and gran came over and hugged her. Gran told her not to worry because she was going to grow up into a really nice lady who lots of people loved and that these kids were just mean because they didn't know the real Alison.

I was quite tearful as it all seemed so real and when we finished I found I could revisit that memory with a smile instead of the sadness I had felt back then.

We then worked on some of the other memories and as they came to the surface, I started to feel better about them.

The following week I started to feel very ill again. I had a terrible stomach ache and the pain was unbearable. I had been overdoing things, which I was well aware of but unfortunately it hit me hard; however I remained positive and I slowly started to feel better.

I then had an appointment with Tesco so they could officially sack me due to my ill health. I was nervous before I went in, but they were absolutely lovely to me, and they have given me a pension for however long I have this illness. I was speechless as I had only worked for them for just under three years; they also gave me a privilege discount card for life. In all this time of financial crisis I did not expect that and I was so grateful. You see good things do happen!

The following day I attended an NHS long term illness course. It was run by volunteers, and, although they meant well, it was absolutely hopeless for me. I had already investigated every avenue I could with this illness, certainly in a lot more depth than the information they were giving. It made me think that there must be other ways of helping people, who are struggling with this illness.

I'm going to be starting voluntary work at a drop in centre for people who need counselling and also at a local hospice, I figure it will keep me busy and slowly reintroduce me back into the work place.

Mark's Perspective:

I think that sometimes it is important to remember how fantastic the resources are that you can bring into a memory. In this session, the introduction of Granny Bald into the memory was probably the turning point. When Ali had approached her ECHO in numerous previous sessions the ECHO had always been receptive, however this initially was not the case this time around, so Ali had to look elsewhere for assistance. Ali could turn to anyone or anything and she chose Granny Bald. Granny told Ali that that she had the freedom to do anything that she wanted and this completely changed the environment almost instantly. Humour can be a brilliant way of transforming a particular situation and it certainly worked in this session.

More importantly the introduction of someone that little Ali loved and trusted into the memory opened the doorway for present day Ali to re-establish a relationship with her ECHO which made it easier when we worked on some of the other memories from her childhood.

When going through this process, it is imperative to check back in on the initial memory to ensure that all negative emotions have been removed and replaced by positive ones. If negative emotions remain attached to that particular memory then it is necessary to seek out the cause in order that it too can be replaced.

22: Looking at dreams

28th October 2010

It's now the last few days of October 2010 and I am seriously trying to re evaluate my health status. The pain has not gone, some days it is better than others, but it's still pretty bad; however my head is much clearer and people are commenting on how much better I seem to be looking. I am certainly loads more positive about life and do not feel I am dying. I have lost just over a stone in weight and, although it is not a huge amount, I have not been concentrating on dieting.

Mark asked me to keep a note of my dreams so that we could get some idea of what was going on in my subconscious. I definitely have a weird imagination. I wrote my dreams down for a week and have come to the conclusion I am completely nuts.

I did notice that I dreamt a lot about babies; it always seemed to follow the same pattern of babies being neglected or forgotten. I investigated this and discovered that forgotten babies could be an indication that you are forgetting or neglecting your own needs. Perhaps I am not looking after myself properly, certainly emotionally I haven't.

So Mark worked with me on some dreams. In one of the dreams I had been working behind the bar of some big open plan hotel. The actor Gordon Jackson (Upstairs Downstairs) came in and sat at a table drinking whiskey. He had a baby in a car seat next to him and he was ignoring it. He clearly did not want it to be there and I was quite distressed.

So with Mark tapping on me we went into the dream. He asked me to step into that dream and talk to my ECHO. I asked her what I could do to help. She said she needed to find the baby and a family that wanted a baby and would care for it, she decided she wanted to find it a good home with young parents that would love it. I say 'it' as I don't know if it was a he or a she. Mark told me to bring in a young couple, which I did and they were delighted to hold the baby and really wanted it. I asked her what she would do now. She asked Gordon Jackson if they could have his baby and he just shrugged and said yes; he didn't care, so they took it and I was relieved.

Mark then asked me if I could think of another time I was relieved in my life. I told him that yesterday I had put my car in the garage and had to walk home. It wasn't too far but there was a very steep hill, and my legs just decided they did not want to move. The pain was in my groin area and shooting down my thighs, and when I finally did make it home I was relieved.

So Mark took my memory back to walking up that hill and he asked me to step into the image and help my ECHO. I asked her what I could do to help. She said she would like a machine that would take the pain away and make her legs work, a bit like a tens machine that would pulse electric into her muscles and make them move pain free. So I gave her that machine and it helped her get home. Mark asked how she felt, and I said she was glad she was home but depressed at having to rely on a machine.

He asked me if I could think of a time when I felt depressed. I instantly went back to the months before I finally left my husband. I had been sleeping alone in the attic room for months. I could see no way out of the hell I was living, but I had to stay strong for the children. Everything was so bleak, the daily abuse was crippling me and I was scared every time he walked in the house; the debt was overwhelming, the phone kept ringing and yet he just kept spending and drinking more and more. There were mice in the attic but I just didn't care, I would lie and listen to them, knowing in a few hours I would have to get up and face it all again.

Mark then asked me to step into that image. So I was in the attic sitting on the bed looking down at my ECHO. I told her that she would get through this and life would be good again and that she was to keep doing what she was doing and to have faith as things would soon change. Mark suggested I brought someone else in, so I imagined a colleague from university called Suzie. Suzie told the ECHO that she was going to be an amazing help to people who had gone through the same experiences; that she would study and qualify as a counsellor and her life would have meaning again.

Mark asked how she was feeling now. I tried to describe it to him, but I could not do it justice. It was like Suzie and I had created a warm ball of sunshine and had thrown it into the chest of my ECHO. She suddenly felt the warmth and the strength and saw exactly what she had to do and how to move forward - it was like having a to do list with many painful things still to be ticked off, yet she knew it would be done. The feeling was like a warm rush inside then it dissipated leaving her feeling strong and confident.

How we got to that feeling from a dream about Gordon Jackson was incredible and it showed me once again the power behind the methods that EFT uses, however strange it may appear.

This actually had more impact on me than any other session I have had and it had a really positive affect.

Mark's Perspective: The Dreams Session

Tapping on dreams is a relatively new concept in the world of Matrix Reimprinting but an incredibly interesting one.

In no way am I an interpreter of dreams but it does seem to me that our dreams often provide metaphors for the way we are leading parts of our lives. At the very least dreams are an indication of our subconscious at work.

With this in mind I had asked Ali to keep a note of her dreams so that we could tap into them the following week. Ali being Ali, as well as keeping notes had also looked into the interpretation of them. Whether this is down to her desperation to be rid of the illness as soon as possible, or if it is just Ali being her normal self and wanting to know the mechanics of everything I am not sure. In some ways I was hoping it was the former because it gave an indication of her desire to win this particular battle.

Whatever the reason, the indication from the dreams was that she had neglected herself and that certainly seemed to ring true. Over a long period of time, she had always put her family first, despite sometime overwhelming odds; finally, when the requirement for her help had been reduced, after Suzanne had recovered from Cancer, her body told her that it had had enough and effectively packed up on her. Furthermore, when she had done something for herself (the London Marathon and the Chinese Wall run) her body had reacted badly and given her the first taste of the pain she now experienced on a regular basis during her illness. This, quite feasibly, could create a negative association with doing things for herself. The flipside to this is contained within Meta Medicine which suggests that the pain that Ali experienced at the end of her marathon was in fact the start of the healing process.

On to the dream itself, there seemed no logic in trying to find a conscious reason why the location should be a large hotel or indeed why Gordon Jackson (preferred him in the Professionals, felt sorry for him in The Great Escape!) was the father. We just went with the flow and concluded with a happy ending and a relieved Ali.

Sometimes in this work you get a gut feeling that there is something else to explore. For any would be Matrix, Eft or NLP Practitioners out there who feel that they may not possess this sixth sense believe me you have, sometimes you just have to trust your subconscious to help you out and it will.

I am sure that you are able to recollect at least one time when you have had a gut feeling about something and have been proved to be correct.

I therefore asked Ali about another time she had felt relieved and we then worked through the experience of walking up the hill.

This memory led us to a negative emotion that she could conquer, that of feeling depressed, which in turn took us to another memory of her husband.

After doing the work Ali was left with a positive emotion from what had originally been a bad memory of her husband and the overall feeling that not only could she recover from this illness but also that she would be well placed to help others.

In conclusion, the path to getting the right emotions is not always a smooth one, sometimes you have to climb a few hills.

23: Psychiatrist

15th November 2010

This is going to be difficult to write as there are so many emotions that have come to the surface. It all started on November 3rd when I went to see a psychiatrist over at North Manchester Hospital. It was a long awaited appointment and one I hoped would finally give me some answers to my condition.

I have to admit, I had no idea I was seeing a psychiatrist until I got there. I knew I was seeing a ME/CFS specialist but had not realised that it was a mental health professional. Does that mean that the NHS are viewing ME as a mental condition? This actually is quite disturbing. I realise it is emotionally triggered but can so many physical symptoms be actually brought about by what is going on in your brain?

The doctor was very pleasant and I had been given a two hour appointment so a lot of things were covered and I was able to answer a lot of his questions. He got me to do a multiple choice questionnaire and then asked me to describe myself before Biff had become an alcoholic. It then got difficult as I began to recognise the huge change in my personality since then. I had to describe how I was now and I immediately got tearful. This is always the case when I have to talk about myself, it's so much easier just ignoring me altogether.

Towards the end he told me that I was in a mess. He had no difficulty in diagnosing ME/CFS, but said that he also had to diagnose me as clinically depressed and anxious. My scores from the questionnaire and his questions had confirmed this, and he felt that I had probably been this way for quite a number of years, however I had developed a coping strategy, and had just carried on. This had had an adverse affect on my health; I had lost interest in my appearance and had gained weight, my blood pressure was constantly elevated and then of course I developed ME/CFS. He described it as me blowing every fuse in my body all at once. The chronic pain I was in was all the hurt and anguish I had felt over the last sixteen years and even though it was psychosomatic, it didn't make it any less painful.

The problem was, as far as he was concerned, that I was taking a huge amount of painkillers. I was taking Tremadol alongside prescription strength co-codimol. Both of these drugs were morphine based, so they were acting as a sedative and keeping me down. Then I was on a mild anti depressant called citalopram, which was just helping me to tick over without really addressing the underlying issues. This cocktail of drugs, although helpful in addressing the pain, were not helping me to move forward. So this was the first thing that had to change. He was going to write to my GP and suggest that I get put on a much more effective anti-depressant. His hope is that once my mood improves, the pain will too and I will be able to wean myself off the pain killers, which in itself will help.

He then suggested the dreaded CBT (Cognitive Behavioural Therapy) and I raised an eyebrow. He laughed and told me that undergoing CBT was not the same as studying it, and also he thought it would be a wonderful tool for me to use. He had no doubt that I understood fully what the reasons for my depression were, and saw no point in revisiting what had already been discussed many times before.

Finally he told me to lose weight and suggested that I join weight watchers. He felt that a group setting would be good for me and losing the weight will also help with the depression.

I had a lot to think about and I left feeling a little shell shocked. The next day I was incredibly shaky all day, not sure about how I felt at all. I worked with a colleague of mine to try to understand what he was saying.

God bless Suzie, she is a damn good counsellor and we do work well together.

It took me a couple of days to bounce back from my visit to the hospital, but bounce back I did. I also made some decisions. Although the psychiatrist wanted me on a higher dose of medication, I knew that I did not need any more help. I had been suffering now with chronic pain for just over 18 months and I had only just got to see a specialist. If it had been at the beginning of this illness I would have agreed but I have come so far with Mark and the EFT, and have made huge leaps forward in my recovery. I don't want to bury what I have already gained by masking my feeling with heavy duty drugs. I want my feelings to be real. Also the doctor told me the waiting list to see a CBT practitioner was over a year, so I told him not to bother as I intend to be fully cured by then.

The psychiatrist also suggested I get seen by a CFS specialist nurse who could point me in the right direction and give me the tool kit I need to get better. Incredibly there is no such nurse in Cheshire and so I would have to go to Manchester, but the waiting list for the one nurse they have there is again over a year, and he suggested that I contact her on a private basis. All well and good if you are working and earning money, but completely out of the question if you are not. So I will not even try to pursue that avenue.

I find it incredible that although it seems that fibromyalgia and ME are recognised as disabling diseases, there is practically no help out there whatsoever to get you back on your feet. This is why I have to keep moving forward with Mark and his EFT, it is the only thing that has helped in any way during my illness.

I have not seen Mark very much over the last few weeks. His daughter had a baby, his first grandchild and I have been taking on clients myself. I feel I am ready to move forward so I have offered to do some voluntary counselling at a hospice. It feels good being able to help other people and integrate into the human race again. People have such amazing stories of survival, and yet many of them do not realise it.

It's Christmas in a few weeks, where has the year gone? I'm looking forward to next year and being cured.

24: Be positive

12th December 2010

Its Christmas again, well nearly, it's actually December 12th and I have just finished shopping. The last few weeks have been a pain in the butt!

My grandchildren picked up a stomach bug and then gave it to Suzanne. I did the decent thing and took them for a day to let their mum recover. Of course, a day later I managed to get it. The trouble is when I get bugs like those it cripples me with pain and takes me much longer to recover.

No sooner had I got over that then I had to babysit the kids again while their mother went to London. They both had stinking colds and were sneezing in my face, giving me kisses with snotty noses and crawling into bed with me. So it was inevitable I caught the cold although I fought it all I could. On a positive note, last year at this time it would have been impossible for me to babysit two toddlers, so things are moving forward.

To make matters worse we had the worst snow fall we have had for years and it was so cold. It took a couple of days until I could get out the house and then the roads were lethal. I don't know whether it was the cold I contracted from the kids or the cold that was penetrating my bones from the weather, or just the exhaustion from doing too much, but I felt dreadful and spent nearly a week sat in a chair. It was too painful to move and I felt I had really had a relapse. I was overcome with exhaustion, had a terrible cough and cold, and still had a really sickly stomach. Even reading this as I write it makes me shudder at what a misery I was.

I didn't even try EFT as Mark couldn't get here because of the snow and I couldn't lift my arms with the pain. Walking was difficult as the tops of my legs seemed to have frozen; I had to cancel my clients and just didn't go anywhere.

I picked up Gary Craig's EFT Manual that I had at the side of my bed. I had read it already but I opened it at a particular page where he was describing PR (psychological reversal). This is what he wrote:

'Health Problems. PR is almost always present with degenerative diseases such as Cancer, AIDS, Multiple Scelerosis, Fibromyalgia, Lupus, Arthritis and Diabetes. From an EFT point of view, it is one of the main impediments to healing. In time, I suspect Western medical disciplines will recognize this fact and integrate the correction of PR into their therapeutic techniques.' (pg 130, THE EFT MANUAL Gary Craig.2008)

So what is psychological reversal and how do I fix it? It is described as having your batteries in backward which inhibits the natural flow of energy through your body. One of the main causes of this is negative thinking.

Ok that's it in a very simple form, but as I read on I realised how negative I had been over these last few weeks. I used to get a cold and ignore it and just carry on. Nowadays I am so alert to any sniffle or niggle I have that I automatically think I am in for another bout of illness.

So I used the simple affirmation technique that Mark had first shown me. I tapped the karate point on my hand and said out loud,

"Even though I am in pain all the time, I truly love and respect myself."

After repeating that a few times, I did the same again with other issues and problems.

"Even though I am ridiculously fat, I truly love and respect myself."

"Even though I have fallen behind on my studies, I truly love and respect myself." The next morning I got up and it was incredible. I bounced out of bed and the pain had decreased 80%. I felt energetic and in the mood to start some more work. I have continued repeating the affirmations all the time, when I'm in the store, sitting in my chair or driving my car.

Another positive in this journey is that I did join Weight Watchers. They have started a new ProPoints diet and I thought I would give it a go. I forced myself to stay to the meetings, which in fact were informative and interesting, so I have lost 9lbs in two weeks and have every Weight Watchers gadget and booklet I can lay my hands on. The truth is I am enjoying it, and I know this is a bit of a cliché, but I cannot believe how much you can eat. I am very boring about food right now but it's time for me to do this and I am positive about the results. Hopefully soon you will see the old Ali emerging, the crazy one that had boundless energy and took on the world single handed. My goal today is to build a huge snowman with my grandchildren next year!

There are a couple of other issues going on which I am finding difficult. Maxine has had her baby, a little girl and, as of yet, I have had no contact with her. Why am I feeling guilty? I had already made up my mind not to be involved with this baby, but then again it is a baby, and my grandchild. I spoke to Suzanne yesterday and explained how I felt. I don't want to open the door for Maxine just to swan in as she has before as if nothing is, or ever has been, wrong, although if she does manage to be a good mother for the baby and gets to keep her, then I don't want to deny the baby any less than any of my other grandchildren. I just don't want my heart torn in two again. I don't know what to do.

So yesterday I bought the baby a Christmas gift in the Disney store. As I did I thought about all the money I had spent on Alicia on gifts when she was a baby, and how they were all destroyed and ruined. I will leave the gift with Suzanne to give her on Christmas Eve. My dilemma is I don't know what to write on the card. Do I call myself Grandma Ali as the other kids know me? If I do, does that mean I have to be Grandma Ali and have Maxine back in my life? Would that be so wrong? Could I cope with watching another child in danger? As you can see, it's hard making this decision.

I am working with clients at the hospice now. It is good to feel I can help people during their most difficult times and my own experiences have given me a huge amount of understanding as well as all my training. Just feeling useful again is in itself very healing.

25: Reversal

19th December 2010

Well Mark decided to try to take me back to how I felt when I was that young crazy person. I just thought I would tell you what happened.

I took myself back to when I was in Cairns, North Queensland in Oz. I had just done a 13 mile white water rafting trip through the rain forest and the day before I had been diving on the Barrier Reef. I was bruised and battered but absolutely euphoric. I was lying in my bunk bed in the hostel, nursing my trophy bruises and eating a bowl of pasta totally happy and blissed out. Mark wanted me to harness that feeling, so he asked my present self to step into that memory and introduce myself.

I think the idea was to get back some of that euphoria I felt at that time in my life, however it was soon very apparent that I had really moved on from the person I was. She was everything I wanted to be; slim, exciting, attractive and daring, yet she was also inexperienced, ignorant, judgemental and, to a degree, selfish. For all her looks and youth I did not want to be that person again; we were not compatible and putting us together was strange. It was like we were a million miles apart, neither of us understanding the other. It is a lovely memory of a time when I enjoyed the fruits of being young, but I have moved on and become wise and worldly. I realise I cherish the knowledge and experience that life has dealt me, no matter how difficult, it has taught me so much more about people than I could have ever dreamt of knowing. I would never want to give that up and the journey I am about to embark on during these later stages of my life are no less exciting.

So it was an interesting lesson for me today and I am looking forward to moving forward and getting 100% better.

I am going to see my parents; they can't drive in all this snow so I will try to drive up to Edinburgh on Boxing Day to see them.

Mark's Perspective:

Psychological Reversal is often described metaphorically as 'having batteries in backwards' and results in negative self sabotaging behaviour.

The two and a half weeks since we last met had been a bit of a rollercoaster for Ali, however, what was shining through was a gritty determination to beat this illness, despite all the obstacles that seemed to be constantly put in front of her.

I viewed the barriers placed in front of her as, in fact, a test and each test she passed was a testament to her resolve. I think that Ali concurred with this and it is a testament to her character and resolve that she continued.

The enforced break had given me time to reflect on the work that we had done. Certainly there were still some negative memories to work with, which meant that there was a clear path for Ali's journey to recovery. I believed that Ali hadn't wanted to explore some of these initially but was now in a position where she felt strong enough to deal with them. However, I felt that what was currently resonating with her was the diagnosis by the psychiatrist telling Ali that she was depressed and describing how this had affected her personality. I decided to try a combination of Matrix Reimprinting and the NLP anchoring technique in order to try and help regain the feeling of 'crazy Ali'. I wasn't aware of anyone else who had tried combining these techniques in this way before but considered that this was worth attempting as it would have no adverse affect on Ali and the results could be interesting. In the end the result wasn't the one that we were working towards but was, in fact, much more positive.

Ali had now realised that 'crazy Ali' was someone she once was but no longer wanted to be. Ali was able to take some of the good feelings of the memory on her journey to reclaim her former self (which in itself justifies the process) but with it came the realisation that she had moved on and that her life experiences had made her a more mature and better person.

Ali was now ready to move on with her journey and leave behind all ideas of depression - a nice place to end the year.

26: Sparkle

7th January 2011

Here we are in another year. If you were to compare me now to how I was last January then the difference is like day and night. I look like a completely different person and the sparkle is back in my eyes.

Christmas was good this year. Biff was in America with his family so the kids did not have to feel guilty about leaving him out. I used to let him come to Christmas dinners just for their benefit but I'm not going to do that any more. That man hurt me a lot, and it's time he realised that he just cannot continue expecting me to make everything comfortable for him.

Suzanne cooked Christmas dinner and did an amazing job; there was so much food to eat. I managed to stay for the entire day, although my back gave up eventually and I had to come home. Alicia and Skye were spoilt rotten, but it was so much fun opening all the gifts they had.

Mum and Dad were still snowed in so I drove up to surprise them on Boxing Day with Katie and Alicia. I couldn't believe the snow piles outside their house but they were so pleased to see us. Mum was in her element and said we had made her Christmas. She was ironing in the kitchen when we arrived; I'm so glad I decided to go, we had a fabulous three days up there and caught up with all the extended family.

Everyone was commenting on how well I looked compared to the last time they saw me.

I have lost over two stone now and even with all the food I ate I managed to only put on a pound, so not too much damage. It took a couple of days to recover from the journey but I certainly bounced back a lot more quickly than I used to.

I have been offered a disabled sticker for my car but have decided against it. I am not going to give into this.

I have embraced the positive thinking and refuse to believe that I will be on this disabled registrar for long, but for the time being it will help. Accepting this condition as an illness and being positive about the prognosis plays a big part in getting better.

Mark's work with all these terrible memories that caused my depression has been invaluable. He has brought them out in the open, changed the outcome of them and made them easier to think about, in some cases even humorous. I cannot even begin to describe what a weight that has lifted from me, I don't need to describe it because those who know me can see it in my face.

As each memory is extinguished the whole reason for being ill is gradually disappearing. I don't have to hold onto the pain anymore and I can see a bright future ahead of me.

I am working with clients two mornings a week on a voluntary basis. I do bereavement counselling at a hospice and I also volunteer at a local drop in centre. It's good to be back out there, and it's a gentle way of sliding back into a working environment. My body may have packed up but my mouth still works. It's also good to feel you are helping people.

Mark came round when I got back from Scotland and I told him that I now want to work on my walking. If the reason I cannot walk is psychosomatic then we should be able to reverse it. At the moment I start to walk then after a few yards it feels like my groin just locks up and it's very hard to move my thighs. I then begin to hobble and it gets worse and worse. It is very similar to how I was after the London Marathon so I can't help but feel that has something to do with it. It definitely was really tough on me that run and I only finished because my mind wouldn't let me quit.

I am too afraid to go walking by myself in case I cannot get back, but I wonder if a treadmill would help. I would be able to walk feeling safe with the knowledge that I could stop at any time. Mark is going to speak to his colleague at the gym; I can't afford a gym membership, but I would like to be able to try to do some form of exercise.

Suzanne and I went for an Indian meal last night for our birthdays. We usually do this but couldn't last year as I was so ill. I scanned my Weight Watchers eating out guide before we went so I would only order my correct point allowance, however my cunning plan went to pot when Suzanne ordered us a Sambuca shot. I don't usually drink anymore, so needless to say I am quite a lightweight. We also had a bottle of wine, then more Sambuca, and yes, then more Sambuca! We didn't eat anything, which was probably a good job as I certainly drank my point allowance. This really is a hangover and I can't blame the illness; I've never been so happy to have a hangover! So 2011 has started with a party and a goal. For the first time in a very long time, I am actually looking forward to this year.

27: NHS pain management

12th Februaryr 2011

Well January crept through into February without any major event. My pain level has not altered but I have been able to see clients more regularly so I feel at least I am being of some use to society. The hospital phoned me and said they had booked me on a pain management course run by the physio department. I was intrigued and optimistic but that changed to disappointment when I finally got there and found I was actually part of a large group suffering from various forms of pain and discomfort. I had to wonder how my condition of fibromyalgia could possibly be linked to the back ache of a seven month pregnant woman.

I almost feel guilty about being negative about this group, because the nurses were lovely and did try to accommodate everyone, however, as it had taken me over an hour to find a parking space close enough for me to walk from, I was tired and sore by the time I arrived. They wanted us to sit on big gym balls to work on our core stability. It was ok for a little while but with no neck and shoulder support I couldn't do it for long. We had a class on relaxation and breathing techniques and then a hot wax treatment on our hands, this being for the arthritic patients whose hands are sore, again very pleasant but of no benefit to me whatsoever.

This sounds totally negative but in actual fact I did enjoy being with others that were suffering in some way or another. It made me think about whether I would be able to find other groups privately that would help me manage my pain. I seem to be able to control it better now and plan my days around being productive and then having adequate rest so that I do not fall ill.

I was never the most patient person in the world and would steam ahead to get all jobs done. I have had to learn to accept that things are not going to all get done in one day. If jobs mount up then I take little steps to get them done. I will iron for fifteen minutes, which is a lot longer than I could have done it a year ago, but after fifteen minutes I must sit down, ignoring the pile of clothes that are left until another day or a few hours later. It used to be frustrating but acceptance is the key here; once you have that in place life does become easier.

Money is a huge issue for me also. The rent on my house is just too much and I am unable to carry on. I get employment allowance and support allowance, which they pay you if your national insurance has been paid. It's only £65 per week and I started getting that in July last year after my statutory sick pay ran out. Then in August, as you have previously read, a doctor and a computer said I was fit for work so they cancelled the allowance. I appealed and I am still awaiting a tribunal hearing. Meantime I have had a lot of doctor's reports that I have sent in, yet there has been no comeback.

I have decided that my only option is to move house, so I have been allocated a reference number by the housing association and every week I have to log in and try to find a property. The houses appear on a Tuesday, but it doesn't matter how early you apply, there is always at least ten people per property in front of you. To make matters worse they have reduced my housing benefit from £90 to £60 a week approx., I say approx.

as it keeps changing by pounds and pence, however with a £750 a month rent it is impossible to maintain this house. It makes me very sad as I have been happy here for the last five years but I have to look for a smaller private rental.

I contacted some local estate agents and have a few properties to go and view, mainly two bedroom stone cottages in the village. I hope it works out for me.

28: Disability allowance

3rd March 2011

Well I will start with house hunting, which has not been too successful. The houses are tiny, which I had accepted they would be, but the rent is huge. There is nothing in this village that is under £650, which still will not help. The houses are old stone building, very dark and the rooms are so small I don't think my 6ft 4" son will fit in them. I had accepted I had to move but I had not accepted that I may have to move out of the village. I am feeling defeated by it at the moment but have every faith that something will turn up.

I have had some good news though, as I was awarded a disability allowance it means that I can have a new car. I had never heard of the motability scheme before (of course I have never had an illness before) and was utterly amazed at the choice of vehicles that were available to me.

I opted for a Ford Focus and made an appointment at the garage. My excitement was quickly diminished when I arrived to find an older woman there choosing her own motability car. She was accompanied by what I assumed was her grandson and his girlfriend, along with a baby in a push chair. It was her motability allowance but it was clear that her grandson was going to be the one having the car. He was very roughly dressed in tracksuit with many piercings, and was choosing a Ford Focus Sport with all the mod cons. I somehow did not think this disabled old woman was interested in bluetooth, Sat

Nav and an mp3 player, in fact she wasn't interested in anything except signing on the dotted line when asked to.

Apparently you can have up to two people insured for your car, and I doubted she would actually ever see the car once it was delivered.

By the time they left and the attention was turned to me all my excitement about getting a new car was gone. I felt humiliated that I was, yet again, asking for some sort of help from the government. I didn't want to go on a test drive and I definitely did not want the Ford Focus Sport, which was the car I was looking at. I opted for the Zetec and was glad to get out of there. The car is arriving at the end of the month and I wish I could be happy about it, but it's just another reminder that I am unable to be in control of my own life.

This is what I am going to focus on now. I am now seeing around six clients a week and it is very rewarding being able to help them move forward. I have to make that transition from voluntary work to actually getting paid, but I cannot commit myself whilst I still cannot guarantee that illness will stop me from attending every session.

Anyway, one thing at a time, first I have to find somewhere to live, which is top priority, and then I will look at the business side of things.

29: Downsizing

14th April 2011

Well lots of developments since I last wrote. I got my car and managed to sell my old Ford to a car dealer which put an extra £500 in my pocket. This paid for cleaners to come in and give my house a really good clean and have the carpets cleaned. Suzanne suggested we swap houses and I actually think it's going to work out for all of us a lot better. Their rent is £600 a month, it gives me a nice new-build three bedroom house that, although it is much smaller than the three bed I am in at the moment, is really quite nice. We have been buying paint and re-doing each other's colour schemes. I wasn't a big fan of lime green and pale blue in my front room, I go for much richer and deeper colours. Suzanne says I live in the house Willy Wonka would like to live in. I've collected so much unusual stuff over the years from my travels so as you can imagine packing is taking some time, not least of all because I cannot move that fast. So as I walk around the house on my daily business I take things off the walls and off my shelves. It's beginning to look empty whilst the boxes in the conservatory are piling up.

Anyway our move date is 27th April and we have booked a removal van. It is going to be strange but I have to look at it as moving forward so I am not dwelling on the decision too much. Mark and I had a catch up as we had been busy recently and I felt I could do with some positive feedback. We went to lunch with a colleague of his who had also had ME and I think the idea was to share tips on recovery. She was a very nice lady but I was shocked that she had suffered from this condition for over 20 years and still suffered.

I'm sorry but I cannot accept that I am going to be ill for that amount of time, I have things to do with my life and it has kind of left me even more determined to get to the bottom of this. This lady had tried many different therapies over the years and when she mentioned the Lightening Process it sparked my interest. I had heard of this and had investigated but saw it was very expensive, as far as I could discover it was around £600 for a three day seminar.

I am very sceptical about this, although I will say that I do agree with Phil Parker's (designer of the Lightening Process) description of ME, he suggests that it is a condition in which it affects the body's capacity to deal with adrenaline.

Mark's friend said it had been very good and she had benefited a lot from the course, however the results had only lasted about five months and then all her symptoms came back.

I feel that I have come a very long way from when I was ill at the start of this book and this has happened due to Mark's ability as a very good EFT practitioner and my willingness to explore the root causes of my condition. It took me many years to be broken enough to contract this disease and I just do not think that a quick three day process will fix what happened over a very long period of my life.

I am not knocking any treatment that sets out to help ME sufferers and if it works for certain people then I am very glad, however I don't think people should be too worried if it does not work, everybody is different.

I have also been walking with Mark and seeing how far I can go without my legs seizing up. With his dogs it kept my mind focused on them and I did manage quite far along the canal towpath. It is all positive, even though I did suffer later with stiffness in my legs. I am still achieving a very slow weight loss, and the pounds are gradually coming off, but I get low sometimes that it is so slow. Then I lose track and over eat on chocolate, however I do manage to get back on board and start again. I never gain weight anymore so that is a plus. Well I had better look at filling more boxes!

30: Marked improvement

15th May 2011

Well I have survived Easter in Scotland and moving house these last few weeks. Everyone in Scotland was so amazed at how much better I was looking which was a real boost to how I had improved. The process is so slow you sometimes feel you are stuck and you need positive reactions to help you recognise how far you have come.

We moved house the day after we got home. It is strange for me and it took me quite a while to get comfortable in my new house. It is easier to have the lounge and the kitchen on the same floor, but unfortunately there is not a downstairs toilet, so I still have to climb stairs. In a way I'm glad because it makes me exercise; it's so easy to fall victim to the pain and not move and that does not help, as the pain only gets worse.

So I decided with a new house and a secure garden that I need a puppy.

I had been looking at puppies for sale for quite a while now, my criteria being a small dog to keep me company which is good with kids.

I had some extra money that Mum had given me to help move house and I found what seemed to be the perfect litter in Stoke.

They were Jack Russell/Shihtzu crosses and they looked adorable. The next morning I went over with Suzanne and Robyn and chose a puppy. He was a seven week old white ball of fluff with two black eyes and one black ear and a black tail, I named him Gizmo. Suzanne could not resist and walked away with the runt of the litter, a tiny mismatch of colour with the cutest little face that she named Peanut.

The puppies are adorable but it took me quite a while to recover from the move. Gizmo had to live with Suzanne the first week and I was thinking I had made a bad decision; I was getting very tired and some days were a write off, I even had to cancel some clients which I felt really bad about; they obviously don't know I have this illness, so I have to make up excuses.

However I did recover and Gizmo finally came home and things have never been the same. I absolutely love him and it was so good for me. He makes me move around a lot more, which although sometimes is exhausting, really helps with the pain as I do not stiffen up so much. He has such a character and really likes to snuggle up on the sofa at night, I wouldn't be without him now.

So I am in my new house and very comfortable now. I am working more and more, I just need to start getting paid for it now. The hospice is paying my petrol costs which helps, to be honest I couldn't do it if they didn't.

Anyway I am looking to start a private practice now. If I spread out my clients I should be able to work regularly with them and I can start small and build up as my health improves. It's so nice to be positive about stuff now.

31: Kick a dog when it's down!

15th June 2011

It's taken me a few days to get my thoughts in line after probably one of the most humiliating experiences of my life. I am well aware of all the negative press there is on people who live on benefits. It never occurred to me that I would ever be in that position and with all the media attention surrounding benefit fraud, it has made 'benefits' a dirty word these days.

I have always worked and was skilled in a number or areas which made me employable. Even going bankrupt did not make me resort to benefits, I managed to work through and set up home for myself and the kids.

When I first went off sick I had no idea that this would be a long term illness and expected doctors to find out what was wrong with me and get me back to work; but as you have already read this did not happen and my salary was eventually cut down to statutory sick pay (SSP), which at £70 a week is impossible to live on. So I first applied for housing benefit, which I received, although it was nowhere near enough to cover the rent. I also received a benefit for my council tax, which reduced that significantly.

Then, as my illness progressed I no longer received SSP, so I had to apply for Employment and Support Allowance last July. As I mentioned previously, I saw a doctor who worked for the Department of Work and Pensions and he deemed me fit to work. I appealed against that decision and was told the payments would continue until my appeal was heard at a Tribunal.

So the date was set for the 9th June 2011, ten months after my appeal. If I lost the appeal I would be expected to pay back all the money they had paid me, so as you can imagine I was very anxious, which does not help with my symptoms.

People were throwing all sorts of advice to me: I should go in with sticks, wear no makeup, and I should act as I am on my worst day, I shouldn't mention my voluntary work and I should cry a lot. I didn't want to do that and felt it would be obvious from the doctor's reports that I was not work shy and was clearly ill, and so I would not have a problem.

They sent me a hundred page document of the case against me, a lot of which made no sense whatsoever. It took me a morning to go through it all and highlight the parts that were incorrect. I found myself getting annoyed, especially when I saw he had commented on how I was dressed, whether I smelt and how clean I was.

The dreaded morning arrived and I picked up Suzanne who had decided to come with me. I had dressed smartly and worn make up as I had no intention of play acting and we were early, which proved to be a God send. The address on the letter was for Heron House, on Wellington Street in Stockport; we found Wellington Street and drove up and down looking but there was no Heron House. Our sat nav was as confused as we were, so we phoned directory enquiries.

Luckily the lady on the phone had encountered this problem before, Heron House turned out to be the Job Centre, (which was not put on the letter) and the postcode they had given us was wrong which is why the sat nav couldn't recognise it.

I had to wonder if this was done on purpose. If we hadn't left early we would not have made our time slot and I would have lost the appeal.

I managed to park close by and we went to the sixth floor of the Job Centre. The place itself was depressing with dirty walls and uncomfortable flip-back chairs lined along the walls, it reminded me of a bus depot, mind you that's probably an insult to bus depots these days.

The clerk came and explained the details of how the hearing would proceed and then we were called in.

On entry we saw a number of wooden tables pushed together to form a square in the centre of the room. There were three chairs with arms tightly pushed together on one side of the square opposite the judge and the doctor who were seated as we came in. I am calling him a judge as I am not sure what his title is and he was judging me.

They told me I had to sit in the middle chair, which was clearly difficult for me, again I wondered if they had done that on purpose.

The judge seemed pleasant enough, however the doctor was a different story and he just radiated contempt from the start. They explained that they were not part of the DWP and would make an independent decision. They also said they were not interested in how I am now, but only in how I was when I made the appeal last September, which was ten months ago.

They did ask how I was now and I told them I did think I was getting better.

It was then up to the doctor to determine my health and so he started by asking me how far I could walk last September. When I told him it depended on how I was on that day, he got visibly irritated and repeated the question as if I was stupid. "How far could you walk? 200 metres? 100 metres? Don't you know distances?"

I felt the hostility oozing from him and I tried again to explain that it wasn't as simple as that, that some days I couldn't walk at all, and on these days I did not go out.

"It says here you could walk round Tescos" he said, "How long could you stand at the checkout for?"

"It depends again", I replied sensing his frustration. "I always shop with my daughter and when I am too tired or sore I go and wait in the car."

At this point Suzanne who was getting increasingly angry tried to intervene. The doctor held his hand up to silence her "I'm asking her, please be quiet".

It was rude and dismissive and I knew Suzanne would be angry. I tried again to explain and was met with heavy sighs as he shook his head.

"It's a simple question, how long could you stand there for?" I started to get tearful, I felt so frustrated and my tears made me feel even more embarrassed as I had had no intention of crying.

"It depended on how I was. If I was very ill I wouldn't go at all. I wouldn't go to the supermarket in my own town so I didn't have to see people I knew. I would always go with my daughter who helped me lift and pack, and if it got too much I would wait in the car. It's the only time I got out back then, I was going stir crazy stuck in my house." I was getting emotional as I tried to get it all out uninterrupted.

He was not impressed and then asked me how long I could stand and talk to my neighbours for.

He clearly did not believe me when I said I didn't do that and again started talking to me as if I were a child, "So you don't meet your neighbours and you don't talk to them?" he said dryly, "Let's say they came to your door and wanted to talk, how long would you stand and talk to them for?"

I was beginning to feel very angry. This man was supposed to be a doctor, yet he seemed to have no clue about the symptoms of ME or how it affected you.

"I would invite them in so I could sit." I replied in the same dry tone, although I still felt tears coming down my face.
"OK, let's say the postman drives into your street, comes to your door and posts some letters, can you pick them up?" he asked without looking at me.

I stared at him in disbelief. "Yes" was all I said.

"Right, I have enough now," he said, "could you wait outside while we make a decision?"

At that point I got really upset.

"Look, I'm sorry, what on earth has any of this got to do with my illness? How am I expected to go to work when I don't know how I will be from one day until the next? Who is going to employ someone who seems fine one day and then can't get out her chair the next? You have not asked me any questions about my illness."

I was really quite distressed then and felt I was being punished for being ill. They asked me to wait outside so I left with Suzanne following me.

I walked down the corridor towards the waiting room and saw it was busy.

"I can't go in there, I am just going to go home, I don't want to go back in that room." I said.

"Look Mum, go back in, don't say anything. When they tell you the decision and if it's against you then just get up and leave. I will meet you back at the car, but there are a few things I want to point out to them first." Suzanne was very angry.

We were called back in very quickly and as I walked in the room I saw a sheet of A4 paper on the table in front of my seat. The judge told me they had approved my appeal. The doctor did not even look up from the paper he was writing on to acknowledge me at all.

I could tell from the judge that he felt quite sorry for me and at least he did have the decency to say, "I hope you do get better soon." and actually look like he meant it. The doctor did not speak, so I just thanked the judge quietly and left the room, totally shaken and humiliated.

As you can imagine, the adrenalin rush did no good to my health. I managed to drive home shaking, then went to bed for the rest of the day.

As I said it took me a few days to get over it and I just cannot believe I was treated in this way. There must be so many people like me, struck down by illness and unable to work, how do they all cope with this? It's like being charged with a crime through no fault of your own and then going to court to prove your innocence.

I understand there are a lot of people out there who are faking their symptoms, but surely it does not take a lot of investigation to realise that the person you are about to see has worked all their life without claiming benefits before and has attached numerous doctors and hospital reports and letters to prove what is wrong with them. Also the fact that I am doing voluntary work on my good days to help other people must count for something.

I cannot quite believe it when I hear about all these people who claim thousands of pounds of benefits. How do they do it? I went through all this for a lousy £65 per week. Of course I would rather be earning money than living like this, I used to earn more than that in a day.

32: Pushing the limit

14th July 2011

My daughter Katie arranged a trip for us in London. We caught the train down on Monday morning and went to afternoon tea at the Meridian Hotel. We then walked through the city to the embankment and went on a Thames river cruise. We then walked back to Leicester square, had some cocktails then went for a Chinese meal in Chinatown near Covent Garden, walking all the way.

I know what you're thinking, how did I manage it? Well I did, although not without some discomfort; actually by the time we got back to Katie's house, having walked from the tube station, I was in sheer agony, but I had had a wonderful day and had focused on everything else but the illness. The girls could not believe how well I had done.

The next day I paid for it. I had to get a taxi from the house as I couldn't make it to the tube station. My body was buggered and my right leg was swollen to almost double its size. I remained cheerful and we had another lovely day, before we got the train back home.

I seem to have seriously injured my right leg especially my knee. I had to really rest up for a few days but still walking was really difficult. I don't regret it at all though because we had a great time, and I did manage it.

I saw a pain specialist at long last and he wants me to change my medication. Instead of taking Tramadol alongside cocodamol, he wants me to stop the cocodamol and take paracetamol instead, then take Amitriptyline at night. I decided against the Amitriptyline as it completely knocked me out and caused me to really stiffen up.

He did say that my right knee was clicking when I bent it, I think it probably stems from when I did the marathons and the fact that I have spent my whole working life on my feet.

In a funny sort of way it's nice to know that there is an actual physical problem instead of 'it could be's' or 'maybes'. I have had so much of that over the last couple of years.

33: Conclusion and goodbye

1st August 2011

There is no doubt my life has had to change, it may not be a bad thing though. I have taken time out to re-evaluate my life, well I had no choice, I was not going to succumb to this illness and I have come a long way from when I first started writing this journal.

I can now look forward to a life; I have a career that is worthwhile and I can now help others to move on.
Life is to be lived and this awful illness takes away the will to do that.

Mark and his Fusion/EFT therapy helped me do that. He came into my life when I was desperate and, as sceptical as I was, he transformed my negative thinking patterns and allowed me to recognise why I had chosen these paths in my life and how I could change direction.

When you're ill you become selfish; not in a nasty way, but you are so preoccupied with how you are feeling and whether you can manage certain things that you stop yourself moving forward.

Once you re-direct your thoughts to other more positive outlets, then things become easier and life becomes brighter.

I still battle but I no longer feel defeated, in fact quite the opposite. I look forward to the day I can go on a trip with Katie and do the Inca trail in Peru. That day will come, but in the meantime let me stay busy helping all you sufferers find your way back to happiness.

On a final note I worked with bereaved children at the hospice last Saturday. We had a fun day, painting and making things so they could remember the parents they had lost. I worked with the under tens and they were so open and brave they put me to shame. They look forward to their lives and try hard to accept what they have lost.

I was reading some stories to the three year olds and giving them all a turn to choose a book. Little Poppy chose a book and pointed to the star on the front cover. "That's my daddy's star" she told me with confidence. "You can always see him except when it's cloudy."

I had to swallow hard to keep the tears from coming and I will never forget her brave little face.

If she can move forward then so can we all. Our star will shine again, we just have to get the clouds to blow away.

Depression

I have been in that place, it's dark and cold,
I cared for nothing, not even getting old.
For poor choices I had taken, it was the price I paid,
For the roads I travelled and the decisions I made,

The best way of escape, was uniquely mine
I would sit in car parks, for hours at a time
People never noticed, as I sat in my car
Away from the world, I would view from afar.

I never saw sunshine, I never saw rain, I never felt happiness,
I never felt pain
Just a black kind of nothingness, I existed that's all
If I had died back then, I wouldn't have cared at all

I don't know why, that I started to journey back
To bring colour to my life, and not just the black
I didn't want to have to feel the pain
But a spark inside me, told me what I had to gain

And so here I am, stepped out in the light
And as the days go by, it gets brighter than bright
The pain I felt, is fading away
But the knowledge I gained, makes me wiser each day

This is not the end, though I feel it should be
I got in touch with myself, and I can now run free
But I will never forget, my time in that hole
And so it should be, it's part of my soul.

running away from ME

A Fairytale -
Ali in Wonderland

My story is based on Lewis Carrol's Alice in wonderland, which involves the adventures of a little girl who chases a white rabbit who is fully clothed and seemed to be searching for his white gloves and watch. She fell into the rabbit hole and found herself in a completely different world to the one she was used to. In my story the White Rabbit is my selfworth and he is very hard to catch. In Wonderland Alice meets lots of characters, in a topsy turvy sort of way. In the story she finds foods and bottles of strange liquids with signs on them saying 'eat me!' or 'drink me!'. She does as they say and ends up growing ridiculously tall or very small, either way she ends up in all sorts of difficulties but somehow manages to escape them.

She meets Tweedle Dee and Tweedle Dum who, for the purpose of my story, are my conscience. She also encounters a giant caterpillar who is smoking a pipe on top of a mushroom; he makes her recite to him.

A strange looking Cheshire cat with a huge grin appears to her and sends her off in different directions, in one journey to meet the Mad Hatter and his tea party guests.

There seems to be no point to her travels as she ends up in the Queen of Heart's garden playing croquet with flamingos with the bats and hedgehogs as the balls. In my story I get sent to the King of Hearts by the Cheshire cat and I become the queen. In Alice's world the queen's servants, who resemble a pack of cards, are painting the white roses red in case the queen has their heads cut off; in my world, I do most of the painting, just to keep things running smoothly.

I manage to escape from the king when I come across the Mad Hatter. For my purposes the Mad Hatter is a 'she' and she has eight guests at her table. As Alice's Wonderland continues to dissolve into utter madness she wakes up and finds herself asleep under the tree where she had first seen the White Rabbit.

In my wonderland I embrace the madness and when I wake up I have a real purpose. Is there a moral? Have I changed? Is it just total gobbledegook?

Everything in my life was good; I was the first born child of the new generation. My brother, sister and all my cousins were younger, so I was loved and spoiled and cherished. I started life in Glasgow, but as my father became successful in his career we had moved to three different towns by the time I was six.

Everything in my life was perfect until I went to school. I was terrified of school and my first memory of it was seeing a teenage boy with strange clothes and long hair being dragged unconscious by a harsh looking woman. I can still see him now, yet have since found out the school, although an old building, only taught very young children. Perhaps I saw a ghost. However my relationship with school after that was never good.

My dad's career blossomed and we moved to Edinburgh, another set of new friends to find, but this time I went into my shell and didn't make any. I was truly unhappy at school but loved playing outside in the fields.

At 11 years old we moved to England just outside London. There I started High School and I did not excel at all. I disappointed my parents on every level and I knew it. Everything I did seemed to be wrong and I rebelled. I hated my height, my body, my glasses and my face. I did not seem to fit in anywhere.

I was out with my dog Shep, lying on the field behind my house under a giant oak tree. I loved being out with my dog and he loved me. That day I was happy, I was not in trouble and had no real worries. As I lay sucking the juice out the grass stalks a white rabbit, with glasses and a waistcoat hopped past me. I asked him where he was going and he turned and beckoned me to follow him. I did just that and followed him through a small tunnel and then fell down a rather large hole.

The rabbit was not there when I landed and I felt angry and cheated. There were lots of doorways, some large and some small, but all the doors were closed. I had to find which door. I am tall so why did I not pick the easiest door to go through? No, I had to choose the tiniest door! I almost got stuck whilst wriggling through, making me angrier and angrier. I was squashed in a corridor full of drunken teenagers squashed in with me. It smelt horrible and felt dirty, but as one of them handed me a bottle of booze I drank it without hesitation. Then I shrunk, I wasn't squashed in anymore, but my head spun and I didn't feel the anger anymore, I just wanted to cry.

With my head still spinning and feeling sick to my stomach I cried and cried. The more I cried the more I felt like I was drowning in a place I did not want to be. I swam around in my tears that had become an ocean, and there, on the shore, was a giant dodo beckoning me to him; he gave me a job and I took it. It was busy and long hours but I liked it and the dodo was pleased with me. I stayed there for five years and during that time saw the White Rabbit often, though he never stayed around for long and always seemed to be in a rush to get away.

After a while I knew I was in the wrong place and then I met a strange couple of characters. They called themselves Tweedle Dee and Tweedle Dum and no one else could see them but me. Whatever one said the other would say the opposite, leaving me indecisive and insecure. They wore ridiculous clothes, were very fat and always falling over each other.

I sadly said goodbye to the giant dodo and continued on my journey through this strange world. I spent another four years eating strange foods and drinking strange drinks. Some made me very big and others made me very small, but I never managed to get back to me. I did not see the White Rabbit often during this time and seemed to have many battles, all the time with Tweedle Dee and Tweedle Dum at my side egging me on.

Then one day I found a home, with a man who was really wonderful. I thought I was safe and I almost grew to my normal self, but one day I found a biscuit saying 'eat me!' and without thinking I had put it into my mouth. Before I knew it I shot through the roof of the house, my arms and legs hanging out the windows and doors. I was trapped and could hardly breathe. I shouted and shouted for help but nobody could hear me.

Then I saw the White Rabbit, he was bouncing down the path towards the house. He stopped in horror as he saw my legs and arms hanging out the house. He then looked up and saw my face staring down at him. He screamed and ran away. I wanted to cry but I didn't dare in case I created another ocean, so I looked around for means of an escape. I saw carrots growing in the garden and I reached my long arm and pulled one out. I took a bite and I immediately shrunk to a very small size.

I ran from the house as fast as I could. I travelled a long way from the house into a completely new world with kangaroos and koalas all around.

I went into the jungle and saw the most beautiful things I had ever seen; flowers with colours and shapes I had never dreamt of. There were beautiful birds and lizards; there were snakes, crocodiles and spiders too but they did not feel threatening.
I slept under the stars and ate the most amazing foods, all the time getting closer to my real self. One day I got on a boat and went down a river steering with an oar. I went for miles and the river got more treacherous the further I went. I carried battling the rapids. I could see the White Rabbit on the shore, waving at me and trying to keep up, but I kept on going, the torrents of the river getting wilder and my excitement and determination growing.
After many miles and near exhaustion I beat the river. I was battered and bruised, but proud and euphoric. That night I curled up exhausted on my mat and fell asleep with the White Rabbit snuggled next to me. I knew then that I could take on anything I had to face, and I slept very peacefully. I spent a lot more time in the jungle with the White Rabbit at my side. He seemed to have given up his search for whatever he was looking for and was content to be with me. I felt I had reached a level of self awareness that I was comfortable with, although deep down something was scratching away to get to the surface.

One day I came across a giant caterpillar on a large mushroom smoking a very peculiar pipe. He was surrounded by some beautiful flowers and they all stared at me disapprovingly.

"Recite!" ordered the giant caterpillar.

"Recite what?" I demanded.

"Tell us what you have done in your life that is worthwhile and would make you stand out from the rest", he replied haughtily.

"I took on the wild river and beat it," I announced proudly, but I could see the White Rabbit hiding behind a tree.

"But that was for yourself! What have you done that is worthwhile to others?" he puffed a huge ball of smoke at me.

"I don't think she has done anything," declared one of the flowers and the others all muttered in agreement.

"You can't have your rabbit until you have been worthwhile." the caterpillar glared at me.

I turned to look and the White Rabbit had gone.

"But that's not fair!" I cried.

"Haven't you noticed yet?" the flowers said in unison, "Nothing is fair."

"But I want to stay here and be part of this jungle." I felt the tears coming.

"You don't belong here, we are all refined pedigrees of nature, and you my dear are nothing but a weed!"

The caterpillar blew so much smoke it engulfed me and when it cleared I was no longer in the jungle, I was in a city working behind a desk, typing away, I was lost again and confused. Why had I let all that happiness disappear?

Then a huge cat head appeared floating in the air next to me. It was grinning like a mad thing and I glanced around to see if anyone else had noticed it. "Hallo" said the cat. "Who are you?" I asked, "Where is your body?"

"You mean this body?" said the cat, and in an instant the whole of his body appeared. "You're a cat!" I said.

"A Cheshire cat," he replied. "I just came to find out why you are here, you don't fit in."

"I know, but I have nowhere else to go." I told him.

"There is always somewhere else to go," he hissed, "It's time I took you to see the King of Hearts."

I followed the Cheshire cat to a bar in the city and there was the king holding court and throwing money around and telling the most amazing stories of the world called America where he had come from. I fell in love with the king and he took me to America.When I arrived I found out he was not the greatest of kings, but he had three small children living in poverty with the evil Queen of Hearts. She liked to take drugs and have parties all the time, while her children had no food, were lice ridden and lived with strange men in their house. They were starved and abused and then I found my something worthwhile, I took the children far away back to Wonderland, and I became their mother. The King came with me but he left the children to me. I gave them another brother and sister and we lived in a fun filled castle where they had birthdays and Christmases and love. The White Rabbit came with us for a while but he did not stay around for long. He was scared of the king and did not like him.

The king got bored and soon went back to the bars while I looked after the children. He became mean and nasty, but I fought him at every corner and remained strong. He just became meaner and threatening, he had violent outburst but I managed to hide it all from my family and neighbours.

But years went on and as they did the worse he got. The older children had left to go to university and I only had the two youngest at home. The abuse was daily and it broke me. I didn't know when I broke, but I woke up in a carpark on my birthday, it was broad daylight and miles away from my home.

I did not know how I got there, but I must have driven although I did not remember doing so.

Then I realised I had shrunk again, there was almost nothing left of me. It was my 43rd birthday and the king had yet again treated it as an un-birthday. In fact, he had never celebrated my birthdays with me, ever.

I started to cry for the first time in years and when I started I couldn't stop. I cried and cried until I finally drove back to the castle. I knew I had to find the White Rabbit. When I got there I took a drink of the bottle marked 'courage' that had gathered dust on the shelf and soon I started to grow. Within a short period of time I towered over the king and I roared at him "You are nothing but a lazy, selfish, lying, vicious monster who ought to have his head taken off."

I took my children and left the king, while the bailiffs had come to take away our castle due to his drinking debts. We went to a nice house and there was the White Rabbit curled up in my bed sleeping peacefully. I finally could keep all the money I earned. I had always worked but had had to give the king my money.

I decided I needed another adventure as the children were older now. I suddenly heard singing and laughter and came across the Mad Hatter and her friends having a tea party. They beckoned me to join them and before long we were all laughing about the misfortunes in our lives that had brought us to the brink of madness. There were eight of us, and we had all suffered greatly at the hands of our kings.

We decided to be even madder, and we trained and worked together and ran two marathons in a short space of time. One was on the 'Great Wall of China' and the other in London. We shared the experience and raised thousands of pounds for charity. It felt good, but it was over too soon and we all had to resume our lives. It was like a loss in itself. I wanted to carry on, but I had to realistic.

Then the Cheshire cat appeared in front of me again. "What do you want?" I asked, uncertain as his last advice had brought me some terrible years.

"You still have to be worthwhile," he grinned at me.
"You said that before and look at the pain and hurt I had to go through." I told him crossly.
"Yes, but look at the good you did. Look at the children and who they have become. You saved the children." he was still grinning.
I thought of my children and reflected on what might have been had the Cheshire cat not sent me in their direction. It was unthinkable. I had seen cruelty and neglect at its worse, I had suffered at the hands of a vicious bully, yet I had done many amazing things. What was I going to dwell on?

Then I woke up. I was lying on the grass on a warm summer's day, my dog, who was no longer Shep, chasing the rabbits all around us. I was older and wiser.

I reflected on my journey through Wonderland and came to the decision that the Cheshire cat was right, I still had to be worthwhile. To be worthwhile to others was what my life was about and only then was I truly connected to my White Rabbit. I was going to be worthwhile and that was when I started training as a counsellor, I was going to help more people.
More obstacles will stand in my way, but my life is destined to be an uphill battle, the thing is, I will never be defeated....

An Introduction To EFT

EFT is a development from TFT (Thought Field Therapy) which was founded by Roger Callaghan but has its origins way back over 5000 years ago in the Ancient Chinese Shaolin and Taoist monasteries. It can be easily described as working like acupuncture, working on the meridian system in the body but without the requirement for needles, instead, you stimulate the major meridian lines by tapping on them.

The creator of EFT, Gary Craig, sought to simplify TFT which relies on tapping a complex sequence of meridian points. With EFT you simply tap all the meridian points for every problem so, by default, you will always tap on the right ones, therefore, EFT is much easier to learn, can be used by everyone and the same protocol is used for all issues.

EFT is an emotional healing technique which is based on a revolutionary new discovery that "The cause of all negative emotions is a disruption in the body's energy system" and can relieve symptoms by a seemingly strange (but scientific) routine.

EFT works by tapping with the fingertips on various body locations. This tapping serves to balance energy meridians which become disrupted when the client thinks about or becomes involved in an emotionally disturbing circumstance.

The actual memory stays the same, but the charge is gone; typically, this result is lasting. Cognition often changes in a healthy direction as a natural consequence of the healing.

EFT is a mind/body healing technique because it combines the physical effects of meridian treatments with the mental effects of focusing on the pain or problem at the same time.

EFT can help in a number of issues, including:

- Enhancing self-image
- Addictions (food, cigarettes, alcohol, drugs)
- Allergies
- Insomnia
- Negative memories
- Chronic pain and symptom management
- Physical healing
- Anxiety and panic attacks
- Enhancing peak performance (sports, public speaking)
- Post Traumatic Stress Disorder
- Sexual abuse issues
- Relief of pain, e.g. migraine, arthritis etc
- Compulsions and obsessions
- Depression and sadness
- Anger
- Dyslexia
- Fears and phobias
- Grief and loss
- Guilt

The Tapping Points

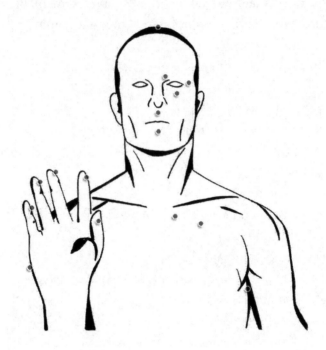

The Basic Recipe

The Basic Recipe is the standard, basic procedure that is employed to treat any emotional/physical disturbance. Once learnt, each round of the Basic Recipe should take under a minute or two to perform. The Basic Recipe comprises:

The Set Up
The Sequence
The 9 Gamut Procedure
The Sequence (again)

Let's look at these in more detail.

The Set Up: This sets the stage for EFT to do its work. In this stage you will rub either the lymphatic drainage point known as the Sore Spot or tap the Karate Chop Point, while saying your Set Up phrase out loud three times.

The Set Up phrase is as accurate a description of your issue as possible, in the following format:

"Even though I *(insert problem here)*, I deeply and completely accept myself".

Examples of Set Up phrases might be:

"Even though *I get angry when I think about how he treated me*, I deeply and completely accept myself

"Even though *I have this pain in my lower back*, I deeply and completely accept myself"

"Even though *there's pain in my jaw*, I deeply and completely accept myself"

"Even though *I have a fear of heights*, I deeply and completely accept myself."

The Sequence: While continuing to hold the problem in mind, you'll tap 7 times or so in succession on each of the meridian points. To assist you in keeping the problem in mind, you'll repeat at each point a shortened version of your Set Up Statement called the *Reminder Phrase*. Reminder Phrases of the above examples might be:

"I get angry at work"
"This pain in my lower back"
"All this pain "
"This fear of heights"

The 9 Gamut: The Gamut Point is located on the back of the hand, just behind and in between the knuckles of the ring and little finger. While tapping continuously on this point, you will execute a series of actions that, while a little bizarre looking, engage the two hemispheres of the brain and set your neurology to working on the problem.

The Sequence (again): The Sequence is repeated exactly as before.

This constitutes one round of the Basic Recipe.

Adjustment Rounds. Very occasionally, you may get complete relief of your distress from just this single round, however, if there is some discomfort you will need to repeat the Basic Recipe, with adjustments as follows:

Substitute the Set Up Phrase you used with this one:

"Even though I still have some of this *(insert problem)*, I deeply and completely accept myself".

For example:

"Even though *I still have some of this fear of heights*, I deeply and completely accept myself"

And substitute the Reminder Phrase for this one:

"This remaining *(insert problem)*".

For example:

"This remaining *fear of heights.*"

Now we will go on to examine the actual points that you will be tapping on, however there's one more concept to learn before proceeding to the actual points.

Finding the intensity of the problem. At the beginning of an EFT session, take a rating of the intensity of distress or discomfort you feel on a subjective scale of 1 to 10,with 1 being very little discomfort with 8, 9 or 10 being a much higher level of distress This is also known as taking a Subjective Units of Distress (or SUDS) level. SUDS levels should be taken after every round of tapping.

The aim is to get the SUDS level down to a 1 or a 0 which would indicate complete freedom from the distress you started out with.

Start Tapping!

Here we show you the points onto which you tap.

First, take your SUDs level on to a scale of 1-10:

The Set Up. Repeat your Set Up Phrase three times while tapping seven to eight times on the Karate Chop Point,

"Even though I *(insert problem here)*, I deeply and completely accept myself".

The Sequence. Now tap seven to eight times or so on the following points while repeating the Reminder Phrase. You may tap on either side of the body.

1. on the top of the head

2. on the beginning of the eyebrow

3. on the bone at the side of the eye

4. on the bone just under the eye

5. between the nose and top lip

6. between the bottom lip and the chin

7. just under the collarbone (in the angle created between the breastbone, collar bone and first rib)

8. about 4 inches under the armpit (in line with a woman's bra strap, or a man's nipple)

9. on the side of the thumb, next to the nail

10. on the side of the index finger, next to the nail

11. on the side of the middle finger, next to the nail

12. on the side of the ring finger, next to the nail

13. on the side of the little finger, next to the nail

14. on the Karate Chop Point

The 9 Point Gamut ...Now while continuously tapping the Gamut Point (situated on the back of the hand just behind and between the knuckles of the ring and little finger), do the following...

1. tap with eyes open...(say the reminder phrase just once, at this point)

2. tap with eyes closed..

3. look hard left and down

4. look hard right and down..

5. move your eyes in a full clockwise circle..

6. move your eyes in a full anticlockwise circle

7. hum about five notes of a song (this engages the creative right side of the brain)

    Happy birthday is often used, but any song is OK

8. count 1 through 9 quickly (this engages the logical left side of the brain)

9. hum about five notes of a song again (engaging the creative right side of the brain)

Repeat The Sequence. Tap 7-8 times or so on the following points while repeating the Reminder Phrase.

1. on the top of the head

2. on the beginning of the eyebrow

3. on the bone at the side of the eye

4. on the bone just under the eye

5. between the nose and top lip

6. between the bottom lip and the chin

7. just under the collarbone (in the angle created between the breastbone, collar bone and first rib)

8. about 4 inches under the armpit (in line with a woman's bra strap, or a man's nipple)

9. on the side of the thumb, next to the nail

10. on the side of the index finger, next to the nail

11. on the side of the middle finger, next to the nail

12. on the side of the ring finger, next to the nail

13. on the side of the little finger, next to the nail

14. on the Karate Chop Point

Your Suds level should now have decreased and possibly even reduced to 0. If not, all you do is to repeat the Basic Recipe for as many times as it takes to get the SUDs down to 0 or at a level where the discomfort is manageable.

Further Tips

Persist in rooting out all these aspects, this is often described as very much like peeling back the layers of an onion. Tap on all the aspects that are them until the issue is completely resolved (you might want to work with an EFT practitioner with this). Sometimes, there are a number of parts to the problem which need putting all together; these are called core issues.

When several pieces of an issue have been treated, the whole issue may be resolved. It is important to persist and treat the whole issue (This make take a number of sessions). It is important to be as specific as possible with the set-up statement. For example,

"Even though I have this stabbing pain on the top of my left shoulder" rather than "Even though I am in pain"

A problem may have different aspects attached to it that surface in the course of treatment.
Drink lots of water (dehydration affects results).
Check for negative beliefs and self sabotage.
Avoid energy toxins (reactive foods, inhalants and chemicals).
Make an appointment with a qualified therapist.

Be persistent, often the treatment needs to be repeated several times a day over a period of time and finally... keep tapping!

7 reasons why chronic pain suffering makes you feel like a prisoner in your own body

This chapter describes just what it like to suffer chronic pain and can be used to help to explain to others just what you are going through. I was one out of an estimated 17million people worldwide who suffer from ME (also known as CFS, Chronic Fatigue Syndrome) alone.

I know how bleak things seem when you are so ill, I know it's hard to find anything positive to hold onto. Your friends and family want to help you but don't understand and don't know how. You feel responsibility for them as well as yourself and this is not helping you get better. You may identify with some or maybe all of the following reasons. This is certainly my experience and also that of many other sufferers with whom I have come into contact.

The main point I want to get across at this stage is to ACCEPT what has happened to you. It is an illness like all other illnesses; you didn't bring this on yourself, you are simply a victim and there is a cure, as outlined at the end of this report.

Let's look at the 7 reasons...

1. You have lost control

You are struck with an illness that makes all of your muscles in your body painful and tender, envelopes you in exhaustion and insomnia. You suffer continuous Irritable Bowel Syndrome and a content feeling of grogginess and with a poor memory everyday tasks become an absolute mission to achieve, even washing or making something to eat requires a huge amount of willpower just to make it happen. This results in you becoming frustrated with yourself and others when you see things either being left, or not being done to your usual high standards.

I often sat alone and thought "How did this happen to me?" I used to be able to hold down a full time job, look after five children and still have time to play. Now it seems I am lucky if I can make it out of bed. This illness is controlling me instead of me being in control of my life. The horrific journey from being extremely active and physically fit, to being almost crippled overnight almost destroyed me.

2. You feel isolated

Because chronic pain doesn't require a plaster and there is no outside evidence to show that you are in pain, this can leave you totally isolated. Your friends and loved ones try to be sympathetic but at best they don't really understand what is going on and at worst, they think you are lazy and should just snap out of it.

This is further compounded because you have good days and bad days.

ou know it is a bad day when you're gasping for a drink, but you know having to move off your chair is going to be slow and painful. You don't want to ask your partner because you feel they must be sick of having to do everything for you, yet you know if they see you struggle they will get cross that you didn't just ask them in the first place. So you sit as long as you can before you finally make your move and you grab the arms of your chair and painfully pull yourself to your feet.

It's a bad day. Your back is killing you from all the ironing the day before so you cannot lie in bed. You get up at 3.00am and move to your chair, take a bunch of prescription painkillers that you know will only take the edge off, but any little helps. By the time the rest of the family get up you are ready to go back to bed and instead of making their lunch, you just hand them money and hope they will choose a healthy option. They go and the rest of your day is spent in bed and by the time they come home you are still sore and tired.

It's a bad day. Even your fingers are aching. The house is a mess and you need to get some shopping in, but all you have the energy to do is alternate between your bed and your chair. You cannot even focus on the TV and your wrists and fingers hurt so much you can't hold a book to read. You feel miserable and guilty because you are making those around you miserable.

Today if you fell asleep and didn't wake up you wouldn't care. It's a bad day. It's cold and wet, so the family decides to go to the cinema and they want you to come. They book tickets for the back row and forget you cannot climb steps very well. They apologise when you're there and you manage to struggle up the steps. The chairs seem comfy but 15 minutes into the film your leg goes numb and your lower back really starts to hurt. You don't say anything, but the pain gets worse and you cannot concentrate on the film at all. You don't want to leave because you know you won't get down all these steps without help. Eventually you have to ask a family member to help you out, spoiling the film for them as well as you.

Even the good days sometimes turn out bad.

It's a good day. You feel you can move a bit better today, so you get the dog and decide to go for a short stroll. It starts off ok, but as you get further away from your home your legs begin to feel like they are wading through thick treacle. The pain in your lower back increases, spreading up to your shoulders. Then just holding the lead becomes difficult and you turn back, every step getting more painful. But at least you have been out in the fresh air.

It's a good day. You feel charged with energy and everything seems brighter. You ignore the ache in your neck and shoulders and start to hope that this condition is turning around. You manage to get the laundry done and cook a meal without too much difficulty. You visit a friend and feel more mobile than you have done for weeks. You get back home and put up the ironing board. You start to iron but two shirts in there is unbearable pain in your back from standing still and you have to stop, however you don't give up and leave up the ironing board. Through the evening you get up and iron a couple of items then sit for a while. Eventually you get the pile done over five hours but it's a huge achievement.

It's a good day. You are able to get out in the fresh air, the sun is shining and you love being outside. You meet up with friends for a picnic but where they go has no benches. They spread blankets out on the ground and you know you will not be able to sit there. They suddenly realise and are apologising for not thinking of you and you just feel embarrassed. You say you don't mind and you will just eat your lunch in the car, it's not a problem. So off you go alone again.

Anyone who tells you this is not a real, physical illness, which I have come across, has been very lucky not to have suffered this, nor watched a close friend or family member go through it. They say ignorance is bliss and that is so when it comes to ME/CFS and fibromyalgia. It is undoubtedly one of the most isolating conditions anyone can suffer.

You know that there are a lot of people out there who do care, but it is hard for them to understand how awful this illness is making you feel. As a result, you keep your suffering to yourself, because you are sure that everyone is fed up of hearing about it.

3. It takes ages to get diagnosed and then the doctors say that there is no cure

It took me nearly two years to get diagnosed with ME/CFS and fibromyalgia.

I seemed to have a permanent sore throat, food and alcohol intolerances and out-of-the-ordinary adrenalin rushes at the slightest amount of stress that made my hands shake and my heart beat very fast.

As a result I became convinced there was something very sinister and seriously wrong with me, yet the doctors did not seem to be taking me seriously at all at first.

The doctors took blood, did brain scans, checked for pituitary, thyroid and endocrine functions, looked for arthritis and anything else they could think of, and still came up with no answers. As a result I could not give my illness a name and felt like my friends, work colleagues and family thought that I was making it up.

I went through every emotion known to man, and I even thought that the whole episode was psychosomatic and I had brought on myself whatever was wrong with me. As a person who had always been in control of my life, I needed somebody to give me a name for my condition, so I had something to fight.

My daughter had cancer and, although it was terrible, we knew what the demon was and could make plans on how we were going to fight it. I couldn't make battle plans for this, because I was completely in the dark, and it was a very frightening place to be.

Diagnosis was the first step and then came the search for a cure, but the NHS (National Health Service) in the UK says that there is no cure! I wonder what sort of message that is sending out to most sufferers? As a result, I spent my days scanning the internet for possible cures, therapies and quick fixes that not only cost a fortune, but in most cases are unlikely to work.

I had to change my way of thinking and learn how to manage the illness first.

4. Trying lots of things that don't work leads you to desperation

As the doctors go through the process of trying different medications, which have little or no effect, in order to determine what is wrong with you, the reality of constant tiredness and pain kicks in. You begin to give up hope of returning to a normal life, becoming a victim to this cruel twist of fate that has made you a shell of the healthy, active person you used to be.

Things got so bad for me that I even considered suicide or harming myself, just to stop the suffering of the illness. This led me to feeling scared at the enormity of what I was trying to deal with. That in turn led to panic attacks and guilt about what I was contemplating and the effect any such actions would have on my family.

5. The feeling that I am being punished for the choices I made in life

I opted for the difficult path through life. My choices led to huge personal battles that I had to overcome. I lost my identity and self esteem through years of being married to an abusive alcoholic. I adopted children who also suffered abuse and tried to help them make a good and meaningful life. I went through bankruptcy and divorce whilst running my own business and seeing my kids through their education. I ran two marathons to block out the pain of my past, and when they finished I started a new full time job and studied an advanced diploma in counselling for four years, whilst nursing my oldest daughter who had advanced cervical cancer found while she was pregnant. I also tried to help another daughter with personality disorder problems who lost custody of my grand daughter. After court cases my oldest daughter managed to foster her and she remained in our family. I finally developed an illness that completely floored me for 18 months. With hindsight, I believe that the stress that was brought on by my life choices directly lead to my illness. However, at the time, I felt that I was being punished for making these choices, rather than realising that the illness was my body telling me that my lifestyle had to change.

6. The financial issues

Eventually, I was forced to give up work and you may well be in this situation yourself. This in itself causes numerous problems: For a start, if you are at the stage where you have not been diagnosed, it is difficult to know to what financial support you are entitled. Even if you have been diagnosed, there are so many hoops to jump through and meetings with people who seem determined to try and prove that you are not ill at all; this just adds to your stress levels and make you even more exhausted than before!

7. Even though I hate having this illness, I choose to keep hold of it!

Yes, even now I am horrified when I read that sentence! Why would anyone want to hold on to an illness that for the most part renders them disabled? Well in holistic therapy circles, they call this secondary gain. When I understood this it blew me away and my own road to recovery was that much quicker. In simple terms, secondary gain refers to a reason why someone may wish to hang on to an illness or condition, some examples of this include:

- *Financial* – those who suffer from ME or fibromyalgia have often had to give up work and live on benefits. Once recovered, the benefits may cease without the promise of employment. This then really revolves around our basic need for security.

- *Guilt and Deservedness* – "I have done things wrong in my life so I deserve this illness".

- *Attention* – many suffering from long term illness find that they receive more attention than before they got ill, therefore, retaining the illness means retaining the attention.

- *Being able to hide from the rest of the world* – For those who have developed a core belief that the world is a dangerous place, keeping hold of an disabling illness means that you can stay inside and not have to face the world. There are many more....

For me, none of reasons remained valid and as a result, I became more determined than ever to beat this disease. When I realised that I had been subconsciously holding these beliefs, I was able to move forward.

The good news

Well the goods news is that I recovered and so can you.

An Invitation to Finally Begin Your Successful Recovery From ME & Fibromyalgia...

Is this you?

"Painful chronic illness left me isolated, helpless, and stuck. Medical professionals were baffled, unable to give a clear diagnosis or anywhere to go for help."

Sound familiar?

If you have been suffering from the following debilitating symptoms then this could be the most important message you will read in a long time...

- **You're wiped out by a mysterious flu type virus** that leaves you exhausted to the core

- **Experiencing excruciating pain** which can come on at any time of day and night with no end in sight... totally destroying a return to a normal lifestyle or existence

- **Trying to walk** any distance feels as if you are fighting your way through thick treacle in a heavy pair of deep sea diving shoes

- **Even the shortest amount of quality sleep** is a distant memory from the past... to the point where you almost believe you are losing your mental health through sleep deprivation

- **You're in a desperate fight with depression, anxiety and panic attacks**... and you don't want to take any more prescription drugs

- You have to forget about the mere idea of planning future events because **it's often impossible and too taxing to just THINK!**

- A constant feeling of being **isolated** from your friends and family who find it hard to understand that your illness permeates your waking hours...leading to even more desperation.

- The gut-wrenching feeling that doctors have **no answers**, (despite running many tests but with **no cure** in sight, and even worse; no hope!)

And these just touch the surface of what is for many an endless cycle of feeling trapped, hopeless and forlorn....

Now the good news!

I suffered from ME and fibromyalgia for three years and have nowl made it back to normality. I believe you can do the same. My own journey and my own counselling training is explored in this book.

But now you can take it further. What I have discovered and developed with Mark Bristow of The Fusion System, is a tried, tested and proven programme of recovery called *Fusion Counselling* which I am delighted to say can now be shared with you.

So How Can Fusion Counselling Help You?

- **Learn how** self acceptance of your condition is the first and most important step to your successful recovery.

- By working with Mark, using and learning **cutting edge techniques** for effective and non-drug reliant **pain relief**

- **Tapping into and utilising** transformational methods of reducing anxiety and panic attacks

- **Quickly and forever identifying** the underlying core issues which may have unknowingly triggered this condition

- By setting realistic **personal targets** leading to effective forward progress throughout your sessions

- **Using our powerful key to unlocking** the reasons why you might be holding on to your illness and doing so in a supportive way which speeds your progress whilst being non-invasive

Plus many other methods which will all contribute to your recovery.

Importantly, we understand no two clients are the same, therefore your recovery work will be conducted in a bespoke way, thus creating your own personal and successful path to recovery.

So here's my personal invitation...

To get a feel and sample of how this cutting edge system works, feel free to look at a sample of some my clients and colleagues encouraging feedback or call and email me for a FREE consultation at:

www.fusionsystemcounselling.com
Email: Ali@fusionsystemcounselling.com
Tel: 0161 435 6311

— Ali Christensen

USEFUL RESOURCES

Author websites

You can find out more about the work we do at:

www.fusionsystemcounselling.com

www.Alisoncounselling.com

Mark's EFT training and other websites can be accessed through

www.mark-bristow.com

Other recommended websites

Karl Dawson's sites

www.matrixreimprinting.com

www.efttrainingcourses.net

Gary Graig

www.emofree.com

www.eft-universe.com (look for Gary Williams free resources)

Books

EFT Manual – Gary Graig

EFT and Beyond: Cutting Edge Techniques for Personal Transformation – John Bullough and Pamela Bruner

Matrix Reimprinting using EFT: Rewrite Your Past, Transform Your Future – Karl Dawson and Sasha Allenby

Joyful Recovery from Chronic Fatigue Syndrome / ME – Sasha Allenby

Introducing NLP Neuro-Linguistic Programming – Joseph O'Connor and John Seymour

The Biology Of Belief – Bruce Lipton

The Body Bears The Burden – Robert Scaer

DVDs

The Living Matrix

The Tapping Solution

NOTES

About the authors

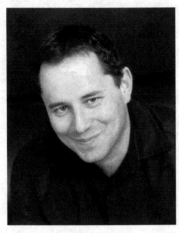

Mark is an EFT (Emotional Freedom Technique) Trainer, a Master Practitioner of NLP and a Matrix Reimprinting practitioner and has a passion to help people and to highlight the healing powers of the techniques that he practices. He has his own practice in South Manchester where he works with Ali helping those with ME, fibromyalgia and other chronic pain related illnesses.

Mark has developed his own Fusion System to help clients break down their own mental barriers that are preventing them live the life they deserve. Mark is one of the first people to qualify as a Financial Healer which helps clients address their debt issues from both a practical and psychological viewpoint.

Mark lives in Bramhall, Cheshire with his wife, three children, one grandchild and numerous pets.

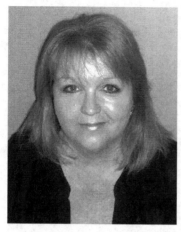

Ali is a mother of five and a grandmother of two.

Despite her illness, she qualified as a psychodynamic counsellor specialising in loss and bereavement, long term illness and terminal illness helping people just like you on their road to real recovery.

Psychodynamic counselling is derived from the work of theorists including Sigmund and Anna Freud, Carl Jung, Melanie Klein, Donald Winnicot and John Bowlby to name a few.

Ali works with Mark at Fusion System Counselling to help those recover from long term chronic pain. She lives with two of her children and their pet dog Gizmo in Bollington in the UK.

NOTES

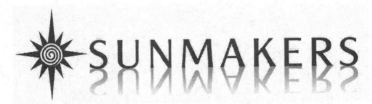
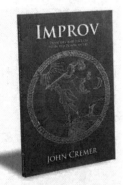
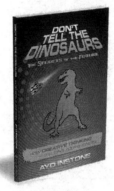
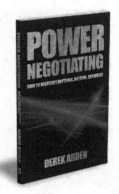
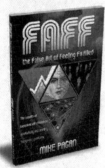
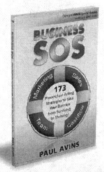
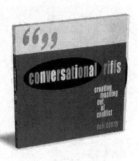
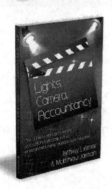
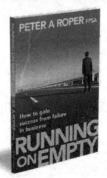
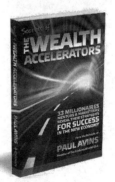